SPIKE DIET

RUSSELL BRANJORD

Spike Diet in the Flesh

I developed the Spike Diet as a way for me to be able to get in excellent shape without giving up the foods I love; foods like ice cream, pizza and donuts. I found something that worked and lost over 50lbs in just about 6 months!

I began sharing my plan with others and they started losing weight too. I realized that the Spike Diet was a plan that many people would love and be able to be successful on.

I've failed on conventional diets, usually all in the same way. I lose weight at first and then stall. When my weight loss would cease, the cravings would begin. Once the cravings started it was just a matter of time before I would cave in and my diet would be lost. I was done feeling like losing weight had to do with luck and guessing. I wanted answers, and yes, I wanted the truth.

So I spent a lot of time chatting with bodybuilders, nutrition experts and reading medical studies. In doing all of this research I came to realize why dieting is so frustrating.

Our bodies are DESIGNED to gain fat and they are designed to hold on to that fat as long as possible in order to survive. Remember, there wasn't always a McDonald's on every corner. We now take for granted how easy food is to come by. There was a time we'd be extremely thankful for these genetics. All of the "skinny" people with hyper-metabolisms would be the first to die in a famine! I like to say that us "heavier" people are just more highly evolved.

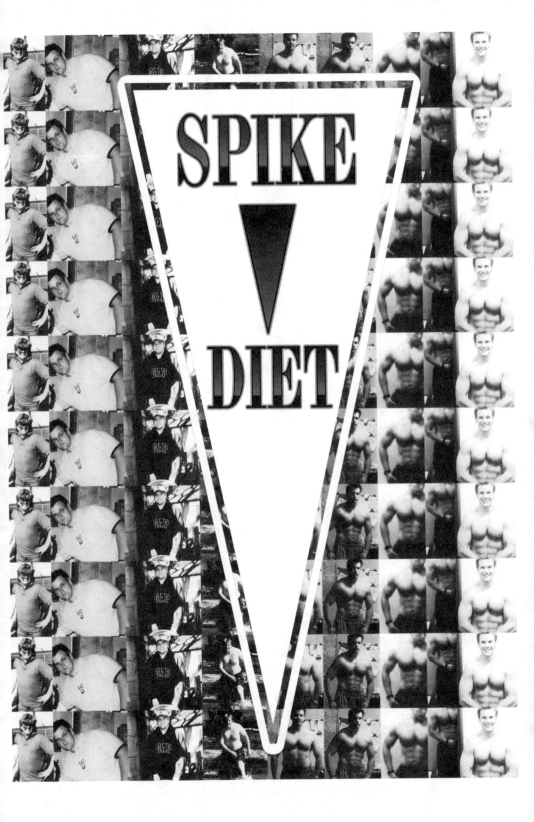
SPIKE
DIET

1st Edition Print 2009
Library of Congress Control Number: 2009910696

ISBN: 978-0-615-32876-8
Editing by Kari Sassaman
Cover Design & Layout: Anthony Sclavi; BRIO LLC, Minneapolis, MN

Please consult your physician before starting this or any other restrictive diet plan or exercise plan discussed in this book.

TABLE *OF* CONTENTS

Foreword

While I can't speak from personal experience doing the Spike Diet©, I can speak about Russ's passion, knowledge, and genuine desire to help people who are struggling with losing weight. From the time we started dating, almost 15 years ago, I've heard stories about the heartache he went through being an overweight child and teen and have seen him try different diets, only to fail. I've seen how being overweight affects his mood and his zest for life. I've seen how depressed Russ became when he was at his highest weight and the emotional toll it has taken.

Russ amazes me daily with his knowledge. I have seen him spend countless hours studying and learning all he can on diet, metabolism, and nutrition for over 10 years. He was able to help me navigate through two pregnancies after I was diagnosed with Gestational Diabetes. Russ is constantly sharing his knowledge about diet and tailoring exercise programs to meet specific needs and abilities. .

Knowledge is power. Russ has shared his knowledge with others to empower them to take control and overcome some of the same struggles he had with weight. Out of his compassion and empathy, he created the Spike Diet. A doable lifestyle change that real people could follow and even enjoy! Russ is now healthier and happier than he has ever been. He's in better shape now than the day we met! Helping people get from where he's been, to where he is now is his calling in life. I'm so proud of the hard work he's done.

Nichole Branjord

Testimonials

I have always been a yo-yo dieter because I could never sustain a diet. I would lose 20 pounds and then the weight would slowly creep back on after my will power failed me. My goal weight is never reached because I find it impossible to stay away from pizza, doughnuts, ice cream, and Chinese food, indefinitely.

After recently following a low calorie diet and loosing 17 lbs, I began to feel myself stumbling. I felt like giving up and going back to enjoying eating again, but then something happened. I ran across the Spike Diet. I started reading the information on it and I just couldn't believe that it actually worked, but the more I read the more intrigued I became.

I started my journey just two short months ago, and all I can say is WOW! I have lost 11 pounds so far, and the diet is so easy to follow. Just when I am starting to crave some of my favorite foods, it's time for my spike day and I eat pizza until I am stuffed. The cravings are gone, there is no guilt, and I am ready for my regular low calorie days. A few weeks ago in one meal I ate two hamburgers, two chili dogs, 4 pieces of pie, Doritos and a BIG bowl of ice cream, and still lost two pounds that week. This diet is so much fun. Just today I was thinking about what I was going to eat on spike day. Doughnuts? Pizza? Chinese? I think I will have them all!

Jason Faulstich

When I first started the Spike Diet©, I was a little skeptical as to whether or not it was actually going to work. I have yo-yo dieted for many years and always start out really good and then after a month or two, hit a plateau and quit. After my first week on the Spike Diet© I lost four pounds. Week two was followed by another 2.5 pounds. Week three and four was a combined three pounds, bringing me to a total of 9.5 pounds in only three weeks! I definitely still struggle with making good choices when it's not my Spike Day, but I am getting better at not putting myself in tempting situations. I can't wait to continue watching my body transform into the body that I have been wanting for so long. I do weight classes an average of two days a week and try to fit two to three walks in a week as well, when time allows. So, with the Spike Diet© you do not need to spend all your time in the gym and eat food with no taste or flavor. You will have so many choices and teach your body what foods will fill you up and still taste good. I have 100% total confidence in the Spike Diet© and can't wait to see what the next few months will do for my body.

Sandra Carlson

I am your typical married, mid-thirties father of an active 19 month old. The most important things in my life are my wife and my child. One day I woke up with an achy back, sore knee and no energy for the coming day. I lay in bed and realized I didn't want to be like this for the rest of my life. I had put on close to 50 pounds in one year, through the usage of a new medication and a total lack of diet control. I made a resolution to myself that I needed to be around for my family.

Thankfully, I came across Russ Branjord and his Spike Diet©. I was a bit skeptical at first, but was quickly converted to a believer. I have done Atkins, South Beach, and similar diets, and while they work for about a month they were just not sustainable for me. The Spike Diet© is something that changes your dieting habits for your lifetime. Like any other guy, I like pizza and beer. Previously, I had been told to cut those out entirely. I still watch what I eat during the week, keeping my caloric intake at my targeted goal while maintaining a healthy balanced diet of fruits, veggies, and lean meats. However, come my Saturday Spike Day; I enjoy all my old favorites. I am able to satisfy my cravings and urges once a week. It's funny, because towards the end of the week my cravings start to build right about the time I can satisfy them, but during the early part of the week I tend to crave veggies and fruit. This is a diet plan that guys can use and make part of their life.

Combine the diet with the Spike Diet© exercise plan and you have an incredible match. I like how Russ has tailored my exercise program to increase my muscle mass to burn more fat through exercises I enjoy. Russ has done the research and lays out to you in an understandable fashion how the science works. For me the proof is in how I look and feel. I have been in the program for only two months now. I still have a way to go, but I am confident the Spike

Diet© will get me there. I have lost 15 pounds of fat in two months! I love the fact that my son and I play all day and I don't tire out. I am going to be around to pester my wife for many more years, and I thank the Spike Diet© for helping me.

Andy Sassaman

Working in health care, I am reminded daily about the obesity epidemic that we have in the United States. For the first time in history, we as parents might out live our children because right now our kids are growing up more obese than any other generation. This obesity epidemic takes a huge toll on our health care system, and our own health. The Spike Diet not only address the science behind how our bodies hold onto fat, but also how traditional diets fail us. Now more than ever we need to be able to understand this concept so that we can change this obesity epidemic. The Spike Diet is a lifestyle, not a diet. It is easy to follow, and you will see results immediately. You will continue to lose weight every week, because with the Spike Diet you never have a drop in your metabolism, which means you will not plateau. In the first 2 weeks on the Spike Diet I lost 6 pounds, and the best part was that I didn't feel deprived because I got to enjoy the foods that I love, on my "spike day"! So many diets fail, because they do not offer something that you can live with the rest of your life. The Spike Diet truly is something that I can live with the rest of my life. Try the Spike Diet, you will never go on another diet ever again.

Brandi Larson, RN

There are four words that sum up who I am...I LOVE to eat! Not only do I love to eat, but I love to eat sweets and foods that are not necessarily the best for me. Because of this, I have struggled with feeling good about how I look and feel. That is until I met Russ and was introduced to the Spike Diet. To be honest with you, I don't even feel that the word "diet" should be included in the title because with this lifestyle change, I do not feel starved or hungry like in many other "diets" that I have tried and failed.

With the help from Russ and the Spike Diet, I feel great and have a feeling of being full more often than a feeling of "I'm hungry!", or "I hate this stupid diet! All I want to do is eat!" During the week, I make good eating choices by eating foods that taste good and fill me up. I feel good with that, but by the time the weekend rolls around, I am starting to crave the sweets and junk that I love. The best part about it is that I get to eat all of those foods that I was craving and not feel guilty about it or have a feeling of, "I failed once again!" or "I will start back up on Monday!" However, after having my Spike day, I am always ready to get back to my "clean" eating.

I have noticed a change in my body in just a short time of being on the Spike Diet. People have made comments that I look fit and toned, which is something that I haven't heard in a long time! My clothes also fit better which is a great feeling! I love that this is something that isn't an on-again, off-again thing, but something that is suitable for a lifetime!

Russ is incredibly knowledgeable with all of this and has been willing to help with anything I have asked or needed! He truly has helped me in many ways and it is extremely evident that he wants everyone to succeed!

Mandey Fabian

I am so happy and I owe it all to the Spike Diet. I have lost 31 pounds! I have been following it and its working even though I am not weight training.

Judy Willodson

After two months of exercising and trying to lose weight, I was only able to lose one pound! That was before Russ introduced me to the Spike Diet. In the first week on the diet I lost five pounds! I was shocked by how much weight I had lost. Not only did I see results on the scale, but I noticed my jeans were a lot looser as well. What I enjoy about this diet is that I am able to eat ALL the food I love, and by how easy it is to follow!

Robyn Widman

I've been following the Spike Diet and have lost 6lbs of body fat in 2 weeks time. I have been lifting weights as a high school and college athlete for the last 8 years and I have never been able to lose weight and keep my gains as I have with this diet. My goal is not to lose a bunch of weight but to use the diet to become as shredded as possible and burn as much body fat as possible. For anyone who's sick of all the crap diets that starve you this is one that lets you drink beer and eat pizza or whatever you want (with in reason of course) and you still lose weight....My Spike Day is tomorrow and I've got chipolte, beer and pizza on my mind.....I suggest you try it out...Your waistline, cravings and conscience will thank you. "The Spike Diet Works"

Mike Montenegro

"Russ has a powerful story to tell. He has taken his own personal challenges with weight loss and turned them into his passion for helping others lose weight and get healthy. His new book "The Spike Diet" is a very concise and user friendly guide, and will likely help a lot of people. If you are looking for a diet strategy that has helped other people just like you who have been struggling to lose weight, then you need to check out this book!"

Dr. John W. Larson, DC, DCBCNBoard Certified in Clinical NutritionWeight Loss Expert

"I have always been active and my weight has been between 133-136 for the past 10 eight years...even after the birth of my daughter in 2006. This past summer I gradually gained an extra 5 pounds. Mind you I was still exercising 4-5 days per week pretty intensly, but my diet was horrible...late night eating, lots of trips to the cabin, thus drinking a lot of beer, snacking on high-calorie/high-fat foods through the day, etc... I knew what I was doing and didn't care because of course it was fun to eat all of that stuff and of course I thought I was burning it off because of my exercise regimine, but by the end of the summer I weighed 139 pounds. My husband told me one day he had been talking to Russ at the club about his new Spike Diet and said he was going to try it and wanted to know if I would try it too. Even though I wasn't traumatized over my weight gain I figured it would be something fun to try with my husband. The first week it was hard to break my late-night eating habit and get used to a lower-calorie diet, but eventually my body adjusted and about a week and a half into it I lost about a pound. The second week I lost three pounds and by the third week into it I lost my five pounds. I feel great and I am going to continue using the meal plan Sunday through Friday because I feel so much healthier, more energy and I know its good for my body. If anything this diet really showed me how quickly calories add up and it taught me to have more self control when I want to grab a cookie or handful of crackers. I can't wait to share it with my friends. I know they will love their results!"

Lanae Wallace

"I was able to keep my weight at 175 pounds for the past 10 years. This past winter I stepped on the scale and realized I was 192 pounds. I couldn't believe it! How did that happen? I work out 6 days per week and ran a Half Marathon in May?? I had an idea of what I should be doing to lose the weight, but I wasn't putting forth the effort. I met Russ at Anytime Fitness and after a few months of small talk he finally shared his story and described the Spike Diet he used to lose his weight. I was intrigued because it seemed to make a lot of sense to me and coming from a personal training and nutrition background myself I wanted to try it to see how it worked. My wife and I started on it at the same time and after one week I lost 2 pounds, after two weeks I lost a total of 6 pounds, after three weeks I lost a total of 10 pounds and now after 4 weeks I am down a total of 12 pounds. My original goal was to get back down to 175 so I have 5 more pounds to go. I've learned to really pay close attention to the number of calories I consume, but don't get me wrong...I really look forward to pigging out on my Spike Day Saturdays and not feel guilty.

Abe Wallace

Introduction

First, I want to thank you for buying my book. I am not a professional author, nor have I ever written anything like this before. I wrote this book because, through many hardships and struggles with my own weight and stress, God has provided me with the guidance and wisdom to develop the greatest lifestyle eating plan I have ever followed. This plan is something I need to share with everyone who is looking to lose weight. I really want to reach those who have struggled with failed diets in the past and maybe feel desperate about their situation. I want to tell you that there is hope. This is a plan for people who love to eat and want to lose weight. On the Spike Diet© I have been able to eat my favorite foods and still lose an amazing amount of weight.

Even though you may feel you are alone, you're not. Besides myself, there are millions of people who go through days of feeling embarrassed, frustrated, and hopeless because of their weight. I can't count the number of failed diets I have tried in the past and I'm sure this is also not the first time you have been excited thinking that this could finally be "it".

The good news is that losing weight is easy; at least it is at first. Weight loss is as simple as calories in versus calories out and a 3500 calorie deficit is equal to one pound. The bad news is that most diets fail you in the end or are impossible to follow for the rest of your life. One of the things I have learned is that if you want to lose weight and stay in shape indefinitely, you need a lifestyle change and not a quick diet. A fad or crash diet will help you to drop to a weight short-term, but you most certainly will gain the weight back when you return to your regular eating habits. Just like a good war plan, you need an exit strategy or your diet sacrifices will all be for nothing.

I've been on many diets where I lost weight initially but, for no apparent reason, I just stopped losing weight. I usually chalked it up to my poor genetics or fate. I was frustrated and was determined to understand why my weight loss stopped. I wouldn't be satisfied until I knew exactly why this happened and what I needed to do to finally rid myself of excess weight forever. I knew it was not a simple solution like "eat less food" or "work out more" (Sacks, 2009). I ate far less then many of my thin friends and I exercised more than many of my in-shape friends.

I do have to take some credit for my gluttony. I love to eat food, especially the ones that make us fat, and that love to eat food, especially the ones that make us fat, and that love for food definitely was the number one factor in me being morbidly obese. At my heaviest I had a body mass index of 41.8, which on the chart would list me within class III obesity. My love for fattening foods, and my inability to stay away from them for long periods of time, was also a large reason those diets didn't work for me. Depriving myself of the foods I love drove me into a vicious cycle of feeling sad and deprived, wearing down on my will power until I gave in. The stress of feeling like a failure perpetuated my poor eating habits until I abandoned yet another diet that wasn't conducive to me…the human being. The Spike Diet© is my liberation. I've turned my body into a fat burning machine; keeping my cravings satisfied and ending my struggle with diets for good! For once I was in control. The short and long-term results created a cycle of another kind; one of weight loss, success, empowerment and positive lifestyle changes.

The Spike Diet© is a series of short six-day diets. You will not be overwhelmed by the enormity of losing 30, 40, 50, or even 100+ pounds because all you have to do is focus on today and not worry about tomorrow. You don't have to be concerned about never being allowed to eat your favorite foods, as you won't be more than six days away from having a day to eat whatever you want. You also will never have to feel guilty for indulging yourself on a Spike Day as it is vital to spiking your metabolism and restoring balance to your mind and body. I can tell you this; after my Spike Day I am ready to go back on my daily calorie diet. I am refreshed and renewed. The Spike Day© is like a reset button for your diet. You know how everyone loses weight at the beginning of their diet, before the weight loss inevitably slows down to a screeching halt? Well, every week of the Spike Diet© is the like the first week of a diet for as long as you choose to follow it.

It is important to set daily goals. Daily goals are the steps on the ladder that will help you reach your ultimate goal. For me, daily goals are just staying within my calorie range and then doing something active; whether it was going to the gym, going for a walk, or playing with the kids. We have to get active and we have to move if we want to improve our health. Remember; you are not going though this alone. Many more each day are following the Spike Diet©, including myself. Take that first step and get your support group together. They will marvel at your continued success. There is no fear of failure and no "trying," just doing. You now have the plan; so with faith and determination you will succeed. You can do it, just like I am.

Russ Branjord, CPT

Metabolism

The most important factor in losing weight is an obvious one, but one that is often overlooked, and that is your metabolism. We burn calories all day long whether we are running on a treadmill or sitting on a couch and watching TV. The problem with many of us who are overweight is that we have a low resting metabolism or resting metabolic rate (RMR) (Quinn, 2008). Your RMR is the number of calories you burn in a day not including any activities. I have found that this is the key, or trick, to losing weight long term and keeping it off.

Having a high metabolism gives you room for error with your eating and it's the reason why some people are able to eat whatever they want and not gain a pound. While they may have a calorie surplus, their RMR is high so before the fat gets a chance to build up and store, their body burns it up for resting energy. For us "less fortunate", getting active and eating is the only way to increase our metabolism without medical intervention. The problem is that most diets restrict our eating too much, and our metabolism is adversely affected. The Spike Diet© breaks the mold of these conventional diets and goes head to head with diet taboos.

What I've learned is that a diet should not starve you and, if it does, you will pay the price later as your metabolism will drop and all the weight you lost early on will come back with a vengeance. Diets that are too restrictive in general we can't follow long term. Only 1% of people who start on a diet succeed in losing weight permanently [1]. The truth is that most of us are overweight because we love to eat. I know I do; eat when I'm happy, sad, to celebrate, and sometimes just because I'm bored.

The Spike Diet© will help you end your emotional overeating and show you how to eat effectively to maintain, or even increase, your resting metabolism while at the same time creating an overall deficit of calories to encourage fat loss. While our body constantly burns a variety of energy sources for fuel, stored body fat is a less efficient form of it so our body uses more of it while we are resting and less when we are exercising.

While resting, the average person burns about 70% of the calories used from stored body fat [2] and the rest is from our short-term storage. This can come from either the food we have eaten or glycogen stores.

As we begin exercising, the percent of body fat used goes down because the body needs faster, more efficient forms of energy and metabolizing body fat to glucose is not a quick process. The more intense the workout, the less fat is burned.

I am not saying we should just rest all day because we burn total calories at a much higher rate when exercising and, ultimately, burning more calories creates the deficit that will allow us to lose weight.

My point is that if 70% of our calories used for resting come from body fat, shouldn't we try to maximize our resting metabolism? Instead of letting our metabolism drop with a flat strict diet we need to trick our body into maintaining and even spiking our metabolism to turn the most body fat.

PERCENT of CALORIES USED WHILE "RESTING"

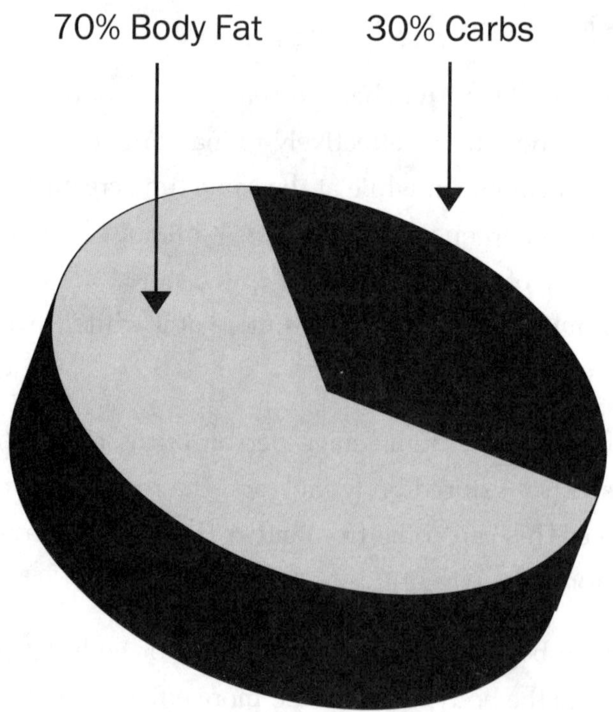

Starvation Mode

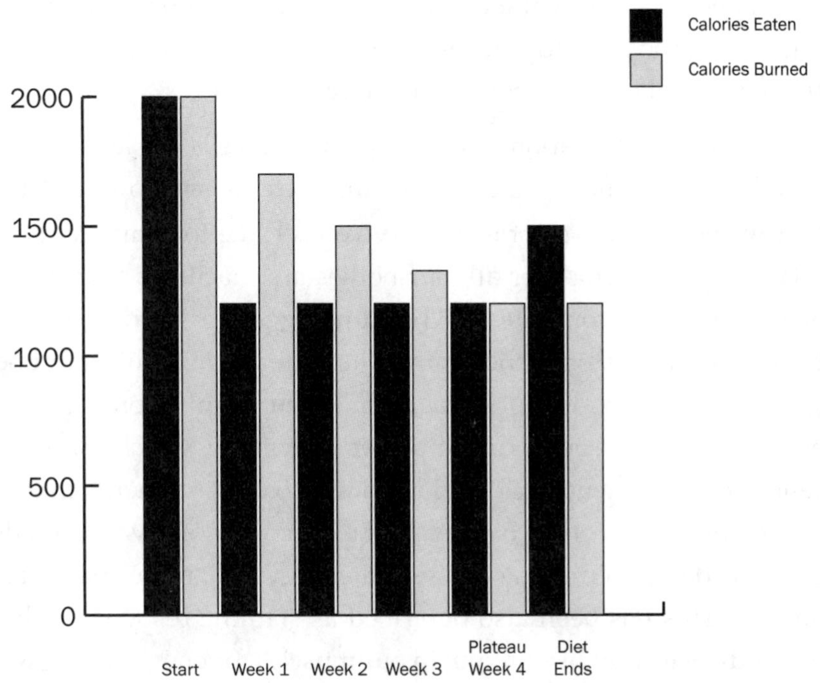

The graph above shows why all calorie restricting diets work in the beginning. Our body is in a balanced "set" weight position; it's the weight we typically stay around and our brains like it like that. Our metabolism is groomed to accommodate what we are eating.

The extreme comes in the form of a diet. When we begin dieting and eating fewer calories, we will lose weight. Like I said earlier, losing weight is just a simple math formula of calories in versus calories out. The problem occurs later because as we continue on our calorie restricted diet, our brain begins to notice something is wrong. We are losing weight and we no longer have balance. Our brain begins to act like we are starving and, since starving could lead to death; it signals a panic response that the human mind has developed as a survival technique. This phenomenon is what I call "starvation mode" and I believe it has happened to every one of us that has failed on a diet for unknown reasons.

When "starvation mode" happens, fat cells are less likely to be released for energy and our resting metabolism slows down so that we need fewer calories to survive [3,4]. I like to compare this to a laptop computer. After all, our bodies are machines that require energy just like computers. When unplugged, a laptop computer begins to run on stored energy from its battery. This is like our body on a diet running on stored fat cells. When running on the stored energy, a computer will run in power save mode, which means the central processing unit (CPU) slows down to use less energy in order to prolong the life of the battery. In the same way "starvation mode" slows us down to prolong our stored energy and, more specifically, our life. This has been also described as "famine response" where our body begins to use protein in our muscles for energy and lowers our brain's requirement for glucose from 100 grams to about 30 grams[5].

Soon we have hit the inevitable diet plateau and we stop losing weight. When this would happen to me on my previous diets I would become depressed and frustrated and usually I'd go back to my big stress reliever; food. The problem is that when I'd go back to eating "normal" my resting metabolism was lower than when I began; and my weight came back faster than I lost it. Many times I'd gain beyond my old weight.

The Spike Diet©

The Spike Diet© is successful because it is designed to maximize our body's metabolism to lose weight. We will need to create a calorie deficit just like all diets, but we will eat varying amounts of calories each day to continually "spike" our metabolism and keep us out of diet plateaus. The Spike Diet© is a series of six-day diets. Most of us lose weight the first week of a diet because we just shocked our body by eating fewer calories and therefore created an energy deficit. To compensate for the missing calories, our body is forced to burn body fat for the needed energy. While this is usually the case for the first few weeks, after time our body does react to the imbalance and it works to re-create a new balance where our metabolism (calories burned) drops to match the calories we are eating daily.

The Spike Diet©, however, has three main attributes that maximize long term fat-loss and metabolism;

1. Weight Lifting: Many women are scared to lift weights; but let me assure you, you have to "eat big to get big." Effective weight training (while dieting) will just strengthen and tone your muscles. It's impossible to "bulk up" while at the same time losing weight. Bulking up, by definition, is a gain in weight. Adding muscle tone will make you look leaner and your body also burns calories at a higher rate while it is repairing your muscles. It takes more calories daily to maintain lean body mass. Physics tells you that the more force exerted, the more energy used and energy is calories so I can't emphasize enough how important lifting weights is to fat-loss.

2. Vary your daily calories with a "high-day" and a "low-day." By doing this we can fuel our workouts, burn fat efficiently and not let our bodies get set on one specific calorie amount. I always felt like I had one day to focus on getting stronger and one day to focus on burning body fat. The truth was the "high-days" just make the "low-days" more effective. On both days we will have a deficit of calories and be burning large amounts of body fat calories for energy. The "high-day" is your RMR and the "low-day" is your RMR minus 500-750 calories. If you have a low RMR you will need to do extra cardio workouts to burn the necessary calories.

Caution: The American Dietetic Association (ADA) recommends not going below 1,200 calories in a day for women and 1,800 a day for men [6].

3. One day a week we have a Spike Day. The idea of a Spike Day has been used for many years by low-carb dieters and

bodybuilders; oftentimes referred to as carb-refeeds or cheat-days. However, a Spike Day is far from cheating; it's beneficial and great for a diet. Not only does this satisfy our cravings, it also acts as a "reset" button for our diet. Like I said before, it's a series of six-day diets. You do not have to be overwhelmed with sticking to a diet and depriving yourself of your favorite foods for months on end. Instead, you are never more than a few days from enjoying your favorite meal. Mentally, this is a powerful tool. During the week when you start to feel weak and cravings kick in, you just have to tell yourself you can wait a few more days and have it on your "Spike Day." The Spike Day will keep your metabolism from backfiring on you and a drop in metabolism is the number one killer of diets with good intentions. **Restrictive calorie dieting can drop our RMR by 20, 30 or even 40%, which is a very significant number.** For example; that is up to 750 calories a day for me and, of those 750 calories, 70% of them would have been burned as body fat! That's almost seven pounds of fat a month I would stop losing.

Between November 1944 and December 1945, the University of Minnesota did a clinical study known as the Minnesota Starvation Experiment. In this experiment Dr. Ancel Keys studied the physical and physiological effects of food rations on World War II soldiers. The study involved 40 young men who were to eat 1600 calories daily for three months; about half of what they needed to maintain their weight. This was supposed to simulate what actual soldiers were experiencing during the war.

After the three month "diet," the men were closely monitored at a lab to see what affect this diet had on both their mental and physical health. What Dr. Keys discovered was the men's resting metabolisms (RMR) had dropped by about 40%, their pulse rates declined, and their core body temperatures dropped [7]!

After the study, the men regained their weight and even put on an average of 10% more than their original weight! Sounds like most diets, dosen't it? This was just the physical consequences; the psysiological issues were terrible also.

The weight gain was mostly in the form of body fat and their ability to gain lean body mass was also slowed. After the study, Dr Keys concluded that any further experiments of this type on humans would be deemed unethical. To this day, there has not been a similar study done.

I think this experiment is extremely important and telling when it comes to conventional diets and why they always fail in the end. It opened my eyes, as I have lost, and then gained weight, diet after diet...until I started the Spike Diet©.

Conventional diets fail not because of some secret evil force trying to keep me or you fat, it's just our body's way of ensuring our survival. Our brain can do extraordinary things when pushed into a corner and this is no different. When we consistently restrict our calories "starvation mode" will inevitably kick in, our metabolism will decline, and our fat burning capabilities will slow to a halt.

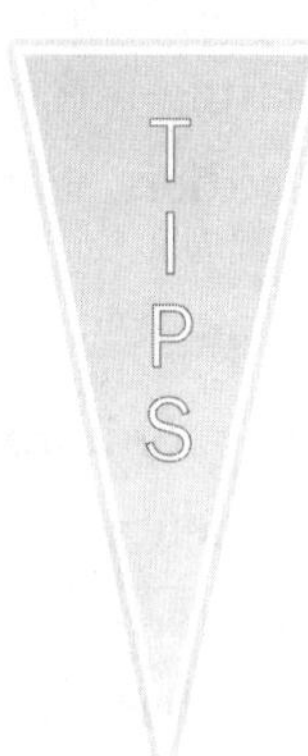

- Eat balanced amounts of carbohydrates and proteins to keep your blood sugar stable throughout the day.

- If you are having a high GI food (pg 40), eat something with protein or fiber with it to prevent insulin spikes and a blood sugar crash.

Become a Fat Burning Machine by Eating More

The Spike Diet© never let's our body adapt to a lower calorie intake. Before it gets a chance to throw us into "starvation mode," we have a "Spike Day." It sends an empathetic message to our brain that we are not in the middle of a famine. Our body then goes back to burning calories and fat as usual. Another benefit is that we restore our muscle glycogen, which in a nutshell, is stored glucose in our muscles used to fuel our workouts. Glycogen is often depleted when we diet; restoring those levels will provide excellent results for future workouts.

"If we can't beat them, join them." I know it sounds odd telling you that we need to eat more to lose weight and keep it off, but it's true. As soon as our metabolism drops, we lost. That's the end game.

What Do I Eat On My "Spike Day?"

I don't really have any restrictions. Personally, I typically stay around 5,000 calories. In truth, I eat until I'm satisfied. I do recommend a simple calculation of Total Daily Energy Expenditure (TDEE) that is used for a surplus of calories [8]. It is your RMR multiplied by two. I think this gives you a good number to judge about how many calories you should eat on your "Spike Day." For example; I weigh 220 pounds, so my RMR is 2,171 calories. My TDEE is 2,171 x 2 or 4,342 calories. So to be sure I had a surplus on my "Spike Day," I would eat at least that amount.

The average person burns about 1,000-1,200 calories daily above their RMR [9]. If you workout on your "Spike Day," you should stay on the higher range because we want to be sure we have a calorie surplus this day. I've had clients ask; "Won't I just gain weight and get fat?" Not really. Sure, you have a surplus and so your body will store the extra energy, but it probably was not stored as fat. What you really did was restore your muscle glycogen and your leptin levels.

Leptin is the hormone that controls hunger and your fat cells. Leptin was discovered in 1994 by Jeffrey M. Friedman and colleagues at the Rockefeller University through the study of genetically modified obese mice. Basically, leptin is a tool your brain uses to let you know you've had enough to eat. It is also the hormone that tells your fat cells to release their energy when extra energy is needed. When we have constant calorie deficits, our brain gets nervous and goes into "starvation mode" which means, physically, that our leptin levels have dropped. This causes our cravings to go up, making it extremely difficult to burn body fat for energy. Our body, in a sense, holds onto our fat for as long as possible in order to keep us alive while it thinks we are "starving."

The Spike Day gives us a "reset" for our diet and we go back to normal, burning body fat for needed energy for another six days of having calorie deficits. With the "Spike Day," and varying our calorie intake daily, we stay out of starvation mode to become a continuous fat burning machine, restoring extremely important muscle glycogen. On top of that, we get to enjoy a day of eating "forbidden foods." Truly a win-win situation!

Another frequent question I get from clients is; "So I can eat a lot, but it's all healthy food right?" The answer is no. I eat what I want and, specifically, what I crave. I usually have doughnuts, ice cream, pizza, cake, cookies, burgers, bratwurst, you name it. What ever I've been craving, I have. I make a list during the week of foods I have been craving or wanting to try and then on "Spike Day," I eat them guilt free!

Note: You don't have to eat a lot of junk food on your "Spike Day." Just make sure you have a surplus of calories.

I think its fun eating the "forbidden" foods while on a diet. It makes for fun conversations when I see people on my Spike Day that know me, watch me eat a doughnut and then make a comment about how much weight I have lost. That's what I do, but it is not required that you eat junk food on your "Spike Day."

I do not recommend doing cardio on this day as it defeats the purpose, and may hinder your chances of having a surplus of calories. I just enjoy the day, I am thankful that I can eat these "forbidden" foods while on a diet, and not have a single guilty thought about it. By the end of the day, I am full, I am satisfied, and I am excited to get back to my healthy routine.

The following day it's amazing how easy it is to go right back to a "diet day." My cravings are wiped out and I'm excited to see how much fat I will burn during the week. Like I said, you don't have to eat junk foods like I do. I cannot stress enough the importance of making sure you get a surplus of calories (RMR multiplied by 2) no matter what foods you choose to eat. Also, you must not do cardio on a Spike Day as it will take from your surplus. One cheat meal is not enough. We need a full day of eating to make an impact of leptin and bring us out of starvation mode turning us back into fat burning machines!

MUSCLE GLYCOGEN

One bonus of Spike Day is that most of your "extra" calories go to restoring your muscle glycogen, which then provides the fuel that you need to have intense workouts in the coming days. This practice is much like athletes loading carbohydrates the day before a competition.

The day after my "Spike Day," I have the best workouts of the week; my energy and strength are maxed out to their full potential and I quickly burn up my excess calories from the day before with a fun and intense workout.

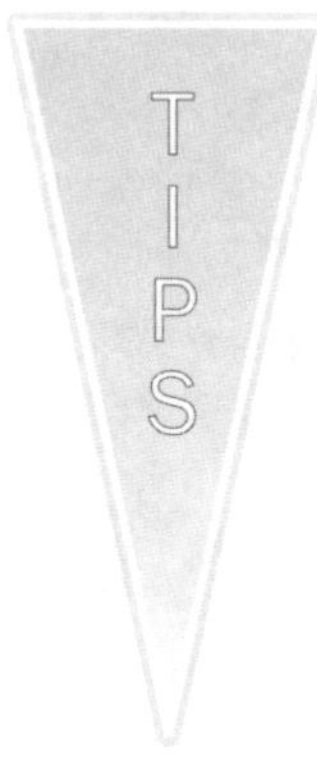

- Drink at least 64+ ounces of cold water a day to keep the extra water weight off.

- Avoid simple sugars, white starches, and heavily refined foods.

- Have something high protein but low in carbohydrates before bed.

- Do both aerobic and anaerobic (weight training) exercises.

- Eat your highest calorie days on weight training days to provide ample energy for your workout and start recovery.

- Get a good amount of those calories within 1 hour after your workout.

- Overeating is a habit; if you feel the need, chew mint gum to get your mouth moving and the mint will ruin the flavor of anything you eat and help avoid cravings.

- if you are having cravings that are not being satisfied, have a big glass of ice cold water mixed with a serving of pure and tastless fiber powder.

What to Eat

What should I eat and what should I avoid?

Losing weight is a simple math problem of calories in versus calories out, it doesn't really matter where the calories come from. If you are a carb-person, it's O.K. If you would rather eat extra meat, that's O.K. too. My recommendation is to balance a good variety of healthy foods including lean meats, complex carbohydrates, healthy oils, and fruits and vegetables. Avoid processed foods and simple carbohydrates. Arnold Schwarzenegger called them the "white death" in his book, The Encyclopedia of Modern Day Bodybuilding.

Simple carbs and processed foods include: sugar, white flour and white rice. These foods are all burned quickly like sugar, whether they are sugar or not. The excess energy not used can be stored as body fat. They can also cause blood sugar highs and lows and lead to insulin resistance. Also, avoid meats and oils that are high in saturated fat; as these can cause heart problems. I choose to avoid High Fructose Corn Syrup (HFCS) as well. While there may be conflicting studies about its dangers, HFCS provides zero nutritional benefits and some studies suggest that it may have a negative impact on your leptin levels; which is cause enough to avoid it. It is not a simple product of corn. While it is derived from corn syrup, it has been chemically enhanced and genetically modified to provide extra sweetness and prolong the shelf-life of foods. It is over used by food companies and I applaud the ones who are now making their products without it.

PROTEIN

Proteins are organic compounds made of amino acids arranged in a linear chain, and are the building blocks for life. Amino acids are what our body uses to build the following: muscle, hair, nails, skin, our immune system, metabolism, and much more. When we lift weights our body needs more protein than the average person. Therefore, a shortage of amino acids is devastating to what would be a successful diet and workout program.

How much protein do you need? Simply multiply your weight in pounds by one of the following:

- Sedentary adult: 0.4
- Active adult: 0.4 – 0.6
- Growing athlete: 0.6 – 0.9
- Adult building muscle mass: 0.6 – 0.9

Personally, I got my best results when I ate .9 – 1 gram of protein multiplied by my body weight. For example, I weigh 220 pounds so I about 220 grams of protein a day; which I find to be sufficient for my recovery. The general rule is the more intense the weight training, the more protein you need [10].

Another great attribute of protein is its thermogenic effect. While losing weight is as simple as calories in versus calories out, not all calories are created equal. Eating in general increases metabolism in the short term but, because protein has to be broken down into amino acids, almost 30% of the calories eaten have to be used in the digestion of the protein. For example if you have something with 40 grams of protein, 50 of those calories will be burned up in the process of digesting the food. This is on top of your RMR and activities [11].

These are all estimates for healthy adults and may not be appropriate for people with chronic kidney disease, liver disease, or diabetes. Please see your physician for nutritional advice if you have these conditions.

Remember to stay within your daily calorie goal. If you eat more protein, you will need to consume less carbohydrates and fats. It is very important to consume protein post-workout. The best protein after you workout is in the form of a whey protein shake. You can usually buy these in "ready-to-drink" bottles at your gym. You can also purchase whey protein powders from most grocery, nutritional, and super-stores; simply mix them with water or milk. Whey protein is the best because it is the most easily absorbed and the quickest to get to your broken down muscle tissue. It's important to get protein from multiple sources because they all contain different amounts of essential amino acids including: lean red meat, pork, poultry, fish, eggs, vegetables and milk products. These proteins are not as easily absorbed as pure whey, but they can provide a wealth of amino acids for your body for several hours. Having a mix of slower digesting proteins are great to consume before going to bed to provide amino acids for your body while you are sleeping.

Foods to eat:

- Protein shakes
- Extra lean red meats, like 93/7 ground beef
- Fish
- Poultry
- Nuts
- Skim milk
- Eggs

PROTEIN SOURCES & w

Every protein source has a biological value (BV). The BV of a protein source indicates how fully the body absorbs and utilizes the protein. The higher the value is, the more completely the protein consumed will be absorbed and used by the body. The chart below gives the BV of common protein sources.

Protein	*Biological Value (BV)**
Whey Protein Isolates	100-159
Whole Egg	100
Milk	91
Fish	82
Beef	80
Chicken	79
Soy	74
Casein	71

**VALUES ARE APPROXIMATE*

Gelatin is a protein usually listed as Hydrolyzed Collagen in many supplements, including protein bars and drinks. It is the lowest quality protein with a BV of near zero. Look out for that ingredient in protein supplements before buying them.

Whey Protein

Whey protein is quickly digested and absorbed into the body with the highest biological value (BV) of 105-150 on the scale. It is the most utilized form of protein having very little lactose and is typically very easy on your digestive system.

It is best taken in the morning, after a night of (sleeping) fasting, to get a quick supply of amino acids to your muscles. It is imperative that you have whey protein after lifting weights for maximum results.

Egg Protein

Egg protein is great for muscle building and endurance training with its high biological value (100). Egg protein was the benchmark for all proteins before whey protein was introduced. It can be taken at any time during the day, but I highly recommend it at night. Take it before bed and mix it with other proteins as it will provide protein throughout the night.

Milk (Casein) Protein

Casein protein is a naturally time-released protein. Casein has a high BV and is often mixed in meal replacement protein powders. Like egg protein, this is my favorite before bed protein supplement.

Soy Proteins

Soy protein is easily absorbed by your body and helps to lower the bad cholesterol. Soy protein is lactose free and is a great alternative for vegetarians.

CARBOHYDRATES

Carbohydrates are our body's favorite fuel source, and while low-carb diets do force your body into burning more body fat for energy, I think carbohydrates are too important and efficient to be completely eliminated from a diet. "Carb-timing" is very important. Since carbohydrates are our body's favorite fuel source, it makes sense to eat a good number of our carbohydrate calories before and after workouts to make sure we have sufficient energy during those workouts and enough calories available after them to recover as quickly as possible.

Foods to eat:

- Vegetables
- Fruits
- Complex carbohydrates
- Oats
- Whole grains

FIBER

Fiber will show up on nutrition labels as a carbohydrate, but unlike most carbohydrates our bodies cannot digest them. It is extremely important to get 25-35 grams of fiber a day. Not only does this help us to avoid constipation, but it also helps slow down the conversion of other carbohydrates to glucose, therefore lowering the impact of some foods to our blood sugar. To avoid possible gas, you should slowly increase your fiber intake [12].

The Higher the Glycemic Index (GI), the more impact it has on our blood sugar [13]. High GI foods have a Glycemic Index of more than 70. Low GI foods have a Glycemic Index of less than 55.

Food	Glycemic Index
Maltose	105
Glucose	100
Sucrose	65
Honey	58
Lactose (milk)	46
Fructose (fruit)	23
Bagel	72
White Bread	70
Whole Wheat Bread	69
Sour Dough Bread	52
Sponge Cake	46
Watermelon	103
Pineapple	66
Cantaloupe	65
Banana	55
Grapes	46
Orange	44
Apple	38
Cherries	22

Sugars Grains Fruits

While the calories from fruit come primarily from sugar (fructose), they have very little effect on our blood sugar and should be an essential part of any balanced diet.

DIETARY FATS

Not to be confused with body fat, dietary fats are essential to our health and do not directly make us fat. Yes, they are more calorie dense than carbohydrates and protein, (9 calories per gram as opposed to 4 for both carbohydrates and protein) but it is just an overall calories surplus that makes us gain weight. Supplementing with fish and flax oil can help us lose body fat. These oils have also been known to help "grease" the joints so to speak. I highly recommend them.

Coconut Oil is my oil of choice. Back in the 1940's, farmers started using coconut oil in an attempt to fatten up their livestock; amazingly the opposite happened. Their livestock not only lost weight, but their energy levels increased too; an effect potentially brought on by coconut oil's effect of our thyroid and how it regulates metabolism [14]. The saturated fat in coconut oil is in the form of medium-chain triglycerides (MCT) [15]. These are very unique fats. MCT's are easily digested, absorbed, and put to use energizing your body. Unlike other fats, they put little strain on the digestive system and provide a quick source of energy necessary to promote healing while boosting your metabolism. I recommend adding coconut oil to your grocery list. I buy expeller pressed coconut oil. This form of oil is void of the coconut smell and flavor; leaving you with a healthy oil for baking, cooking and frying. I use it in place of regular cooking oil when making things like oatmeal waffles, or in place of butter for bread and baking.

Foods to eat:

- Nuts
- Healthy un-refined oils
- Coconut oil

EAT FOR BALANCE

For individuals who exercise and lift weights on a regular basis on the Spike Diet©, I recommend a balanced amount of macronutrients when it comes to carbohydrates and protein; and a lesser amount of dietary fat. A good calorie split is 40% from carbohydrates, 40% from protein, and 20% from fat. I feel this is a good average but doesn't need to be followed perfectly.

The chart below shows you a good goal of macronutrients to aim for daily based on the amount of calories you eat. The chart is for both men and women who are lifting weights 3-5 times a week.

Calories	Fat 20%	Carbs 40 %	Protein 40%
1200	27 grams	120 grams	120 grams
1500	33 grams	150 grams	150 grams
1750	39 grams	175 grams	175 grams
2000	44 grams	200 grams	200 grams
2500	56 grams	250 grams	250 grams

For the men and women who are not lifting weights, you will not need as much protein.

Calories	Fat 20%	Carbs 60 %	Protein 20%
1200	27 grams	180 grams	60 grams
1500	33 grams	225 grams	75 grams
1750	39 grams	262 grams	88 grams
2000	44 grams	300 grams	100 grams
2500	56 grams	375 grams	125 grams

CALORIE TIMING

The truth is a strong diet will have a good balance of protein, carbohydrates, and fats. The timing of those calories can be extremely beneficial to your progress. For example; since carbohydrates are our body's preferred energy source, we should eat them when we plan on needing energy, i.e. lifting weights, on our way to work, or for activities like hiking and biking. Night time is a great time to up your dietary fat as the fats are slowly digested which will help fuel your body as you sleep and help save your lean body mass as you spend several hours fasting. Protein is a must in the morning after you break your fast, because your body may be scavenging your muscles for any amino acids it may be lacking. Protein is also an absolute requirement immediately after you lift weights. Not eating protein after lifting weights is like filling a bath tub without plugging the drain. You'll get nowhere. All of the hard work you put into your workout will be wasted. Also, to ensure my body is always in a positive nitrogen balance, meaning it has amino acids available to use when it needs to, I eat something with 15+ grams of protein in each day of my 6 meals about every two-three hours and slow-digesting protein before bed.

Food to Eat

- Lean Meats
- Fish
- Poultry
- Protein Powders
- Beans and Legumes
- Eggs
- Nuts
- Skim Milk
- Reduced Fat Cheese
- Vegetables
- Fruits
- Oats
- Whole Grains
- Quinoa
- Olive Oil
- Coconut Oil

Foods to Avoid

- Sugar
- White Bread
- White Pasta
- Vegetable Oil
- Butter
- Shortening
- Whole Milk
- Whole Fat Cheese
- Processed Foods
- Cereals High in Sugar
- HFCS

Getting Started with Your RMR

When you get started on your Spike Diet©, you will need to use the formula below to get an estimate of your resting metabolic rate (RMR), also referred to as your basal metabolic rate (BMR), as we use that as the base for your daily calorie intake. I use (RMR) resting metabolic rate because I believe it creates less confusion. This is a chart based of the Harris and Benedict Formula [16].

Harris and Benedict RMR Formula:

Women: RMR = 655 + (4.35 x weight in pounds) + (4.7 x height in inches) – 4.7 x age in years)

Men: RMR = 66 + (6.23 x weight in pounds) + (12.7 x height in inches) – (6.8 x age in years)

For example; Rose is a woman that is 5'3" and weighs 160 pounds and is 35 years old. Her formula would be:

655 + (4.35 x 160) 1,351 + (4.7 x 63) 296.1
– (4.7 x 35) 164.5 = 1,482.6 calories

For Rose to lose weight, she needs to eat fewer calories and/or burn calories through exercise to be under her RMR of 1,482.6.

When I started this diet, I was 265 pounds, 6'3" and 32 years old; using the formula or men, my RMR looked like this:

RMR = 66 + (6.23 x 265) + (12.7 x 75)
– (6.8 x 32) = 2,454 calories

Your RMR is the starting point for your daily calorie goal.

"High Calorie Days" is your RMR. My goal is 2,454 calories per day.

"Low Calorie Days" is your RMR minus 500 calories.

It is best to exercise on your "high days" as you have more energy available for your workouts and recovery.

Spike Day is your RMR x's 2.

You can have two to three "high-days" in a week. Your "low-day" is your RMR calories minus 500-700 calories. I recommend you do not go below 1,200 calories a day [17]. If your "low-day" puts you below 1,200 calories, you should stop there and do a bit more cardio to make up the difference. For example; if your RMR is 1,300, subtracting 500 calories would give you 800 for your daily allowance. So eat 1,200 and burn an extra 400 with cardio. This is where having some extra lean body mass will come in handy as that will raise your RMR.

Your Spike Day is your RMR multiplied by 2, which defines a calorie surplus based on using your Total Daily Energy Expenditure (TDEE), and activity multiplier.

Activity Multiplier

Sedentary = RMR x 1.2
(little or no exercise / activity)
Lightly active = RMR x 1.375
(exercise and activity 1-3 days per week)
Moderately active = RMR x 1.55
(exercise and activity 3-5 days per week)
Very active = RMR x 1.725
(exercise and activity 6-7 days per week)
Extremely active = RMR x 1.9
(daily exercise or physical job)

Calorie surplus = RMR x 2

Remember to log your calories and workouts; this is extremely important to making and maintaining your progress. This is the history and action plan of your diet, and if there's a problem, it will show in your logs. I've had many people realize that they were eating too little after they started logging their meals. It also lets you know what you can have for dinner or a night-time snack. I know it's tedious, but this is too important to not take the time to do.

A sample week on the Spike Diet©

DAY	Sunday	Monday	Tuesday	Wednesday	Thursday	Friday	Saturday
CALORIE GOAL	High-Day	Low-Day	Low-Day	High-Day	High-Day	Low-Day	SPIKE DAY!
EXERCISE	Upper Body	Cardio	Cardio	Lower Body	Upper Body	Cardio	NONE

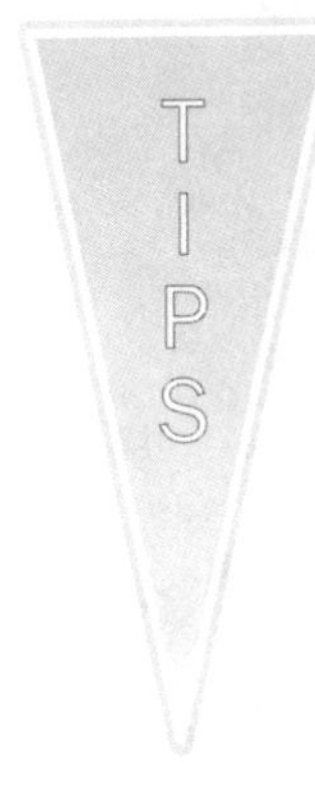

• 90% of our Growth Hormone supply is released while we sleep, and not only does (GH) it help us build muscle, it is also key for burning fat for energy.

• Dietary fat in moderation is fine; make sure you get your essential fats including Omega-3 and Omega-6.

• Eat 6-8 small meals a day to keep your metabolism high and cravings down.

• Begin each morning with a glass of ice water to kick start your metabolism.

• Supplement your diet with purified enteric coated fish oil caps to get your essential fats without the fishy after taste.

• 3500 callories of a surplus or a deficit equals 1 pound gained or lost.

• Buy a pedometer and get moving: walking and moving every hour of everyday will give your metabolism an extra boost to help you burn body fat for energy. Set a goal for 10,000 steps everyday

The Spike Diet© by Numbers

Here's how math can show you how you lose weight on the Spike Diet©. You should put in your numbers to see what you can expect to lose a week on the Spike Diet©.

My RMR is 2,500 calories, which is what I burn a day not including activities. Using the "activity multiplier," I exercise about three to four days a week, so that would make me "moderately active" with a 1.55 multiplier. I burn on average 2,500 calories x 1.55 or 3,750 calories a day and 26,250 calories each week.

Example 1

My "high-day" food intake is my RMR calories three days a week:

2,500 x 3 = 7,500 calories.

On the three other "low-days" I eat 2,000 calories;

2,000 x 3 = 6,000 calories

On my Spike Day I eat 2,500 x 2 which equals 5,000 calories.

So for the week, I ate 18,500 total calories. My deficit for the week is 26,250 subtract 18,500 which nets me a negative 7,750 calories. Since one pound is equal to 3,500 calories, I divide my deficit by 3,500; 7,750 divided by 3,500 which equals a loss of 2.2 pounds!

Example 2

Here's an example of a woman who weighs 175 pounds and her RMR is 1,600 calories. She exercises three days a week, so her multiplier is 1.55.

1,600 x 1.55 (activity multiplier) = 2,480 calories burned daily and 17,360 per week.

1,600 calories eaten three days a week, or 4,800 total

1,200 calories eaten three days a week, or 3,600 total

On her "Spike Day," she eats 1,600 x 2 or 3,200 calories.

Her total burned = 17,360 calories

Total consumed = 11,600 calories

Her deficit = 5,760 and that divided by 3,500 equals 1.65 pounds lost per week.

You have *six* days of a calorie deficit where your body will need to burn extra body fat for energy, and one day of a surplus to keep your metabolism honest.

The average person should lose about two pounds each week on this diet. Two pounds a week is outstanding when you figure that's 104 pounds in a year! This is not a fad or crash diet. It's not about how much you lose in one week, but what you lose during the diet and keep off for good.

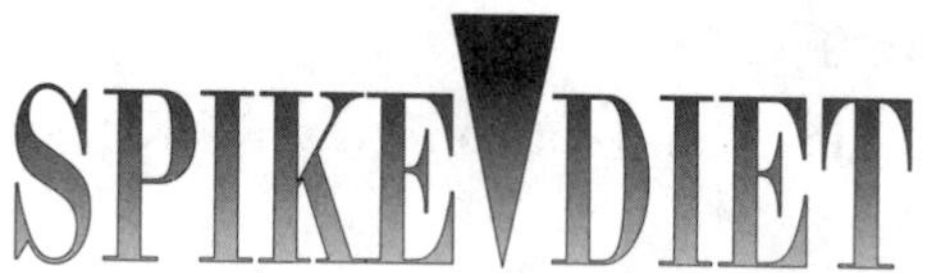

QUICK START GUIDE

Height in Inches	Weight in Pounds	Age

Harris and Benedict RMR Formula

Women: RMR=655+(4.35 x weight in pounds) + (4.7 x height in inches) - (4.7 x age in years)
Men: RMR=66+(6.23 x weight in pounds) + (12.7 x height in inches) - (6.8 x age in years)

RMR=	

Daily Resting Calories burned-High Day	RMR		X 3= Weekly Calories on a High Day
Low Day	RMR - 500		X 3= Weekly Calories on a Low Day
SPIKE DAY	RMR X 2		
Average Total Calories Burned with Activity	(TDEE)= RMR X 1.55		X 7= Weekly Calories Burned

Activity Multiplier for TDEE

Sedentary=RMR x 1.2 (little or no exercise or activity)
Lightly Active=RMR x 1.375 (exercise and activity 1-3 days/wk)
Moderately Active=RMR x 1.55 (exercise and activity 3-5 days/wk)
Very Active=RMR x 1.725 (exercise and activity 6-7 days/wk)
Extremely Active=RMR x 1.9 (daily exercise or physical job)

Total Calories Burned	Total Calories Consumed	Burned-Consumed =(Deficit)	Divide Deficit by 3500 (1lb)	Pounds lost per week

WORKOUTS

For workouts I use split-body workouts. For example; I have three lifting days each week, but I change up the splits periodically to keep things fresh.

Days 1-3	Part A	Part B
Day 1	Chest & Triceps	Chest & Back
Day 2	Back, Biceps & Abdominal Muscles	Biceps, Triceps & Shoulders
Day 3	Legs & Shoulders	Legs & Abdominal Muscles

Feel free to experiment with your own splits as the effectiveness of workouts can vary greatly depending on everyone's own personal preference. Keeping yourself excited and motivated to keep working out is the most important part.

Some of my favorite workout routines are:

(1) High Volume Training

(2) Max-OT – a program designed around quick intense workouts

(3) High Intensity Training or HIT, developed by Mike Mentzer

(4) Pyramid Training

Note: It is extremely important to use a spotter with this and all exercises from the programs I have listed, but especially the ones in which you are lifting "heavy" weights.

HIGH VOLUME TRAINING

High volume training could be described as a great and simple beginner's routine. The workout involves about 12 sets per body part. Repetitions range from 10 – 12 per exercise. Below is an example of a workout using the high volume training program.

Day 1A: Here you are training chest and triceps. I chose those two body parts because most of the compound exercises you do work both groups since they compliment each other. Compound exercises will hit multiple body parts, so when you are counting sets; you have to factor that in. For example, a bench press hits both your (pectoral muscles) chest and your triceps (back of your arms), so that would be one exercise for both. If you complete three sets, you just did three sets of each so now you need nine more sets of chest and nine more of triceps.

Isolation exercises only hit one muscle group. An example of an isolated chest movement is cable cross-over and an example of an isolated triceps movement is a triceps rope extensions.

The table below is a simplified example of a chest and triceps workout that will give you 12 sets per body part.

EXERCISE	SET 1	SET 2	SET 3
Flat Bench Press (Chest & Triceps)			
Incline Bench Press (Chest & Triceps)			
Dips (Chest & Triceps)			
Triceps Rope Extension (Triceps)			
Cable Crossover (Chest)			

MAX-OT

Max-OT is a lifting program designed around short and intense workouts [18]. It involves six to nine sets per body part that are done in the four to six repetition ranges. The last repetition of every exercise is done to exhaustion, meaning to the point you can not do anymore. The workouts are very short. You should complete a full workout in 30-45 minutes. Give yourself a rest period of about two to three minutes between sets. Max-OT combines heavy weights with low repetitions. The website says it can be done by beginners, I recommend this workout be done by people who have experience in weight training or under the supervision of a personal trainer.

HIGH INTENSITY TRAINING (HIT)

Developed by one of bodybuilding's true legends, Mike Mentzer, this program is also focused on short intense workouts [19]. HIT is even shorter than Max-OT and requires four to seven days off between workouts. I like this technique because it nails the basic principle of muscle building; which is force your body to adapt to a workload it can't handle by going to exhaustion on short workouts and then let the real magic happen with proper rest and recovery.

PYRAMID TRAINING

Pyramid weight training is what I learned growing up playing football. It is based on high repetitions moving up to lower repetitions as the workout progressed. A typical lifting pyramid involves six to eight sets, beginning with lighter weights and high repetitions moving toward heavier weights and fewer repetitions.

1) 15 Repetitions
2) 12 Repetitions
3) 10 Repetitions
4) 8 Repetitions
5) 6 Repetitions
6) 4 Repetitions

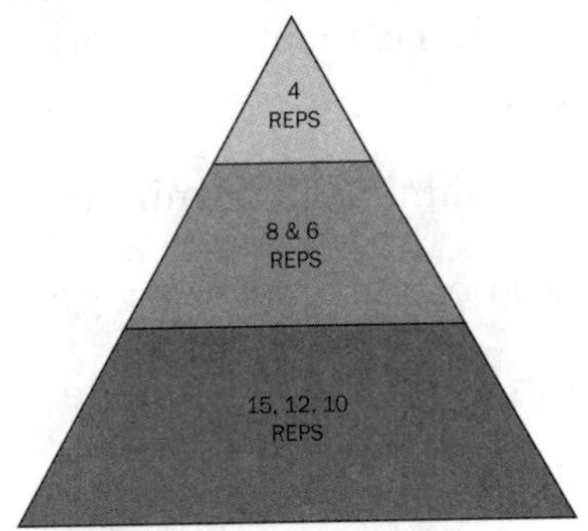

The problem I have with this type of training is you are usually fatigued when you get to the higher weights where I think you want to be at your strongest point to get muscle growth. Some weight lifters love this workout and it is similar to high volume training with many sets and repetitions.

JOIN A GYM

A gym membership can be as cheap as $1.00 a day…a very worthwhile investment. I know from past experience that it can be extremely difficult to have efficient workouts at home. Also, if you have limited knowledge of workouts, I highly recommend you hire a personal trainer. You will be beginning a new lifestyle and becoming a new person and that new person is really going to enjoy working out. Don't be intimidated by a gym or its members; we all have to start somewhere. I commend you for the courage it takes to walk into a gym for the first time despite any fears you may have.

Remember to drink a whey protein shake immediately following your weight training: 40 grams for men and 20-30 grams for women. If you are doing cardio after your weight lifting, make sure you drink your shake before doing cardio. It is more effective to lift weights before a cardio workout; otherwise you will burn the fuel you need for your weight lifting.

Ideally, your workout days should go like this:

(1) Warm-up. Eat something small before lifting like a banana. It should be about 100 calories full of good healthy carbohydrates.

(2) Weight training 30-45 minutes

(3) Have a post workout whey protein shake

(4) Cardio workout 30-45 minutes

(5) Meal

The best time to do a cardio workout is in the morning, before eating carbohydrates. You will have less stored and you body will need to burn more body-fat to fuel your workout.

The fat-burning zone is a low intensity workout. As your heart-rate increases, body-fat is extremely difficult to metabolize for energy, so keeping it below 140 beats per minute, burns a higher percentage of body-fat than a cardio zone. But, keep in mind you actually burn more calories overall in the cardio zone.

Another great type of cardio workout to burn body-fat is High Intensity Interval Training (HIIT); which is 30 second intervals of high intensity cardio, like sprinting, followed by 30 seconds of low intensity like walking or jogging [20]. Do the 30 second intervals of fast then slow for 8-15 minutes. This type of exercise is great because it burns a lot of calories after the fact with a metabolism boost.

SUPPLEMENTS 101

Whey Protein

Whey Protein is the most important supplement to gain strength and lean muscle mass. It has the highest biological value (BV) of any protein. This means it is the most easily absorbed and used. It is extremely important to get 20-40 grams immediately following a workout and, if possible, first thing in the morning because your body just spent several hours fasting while you were sleeping.

Creatine Monohydrate and other types of Creatine

- Creatine fuels ATP development
- Sustained high intensity and power workouts
- More energy for muscle contraction
- Vastly improved power and muscle size
- You workout longer, stronger and get to see the results in the mirror.
- Many pre-workout supplements include Creatine with Arginine to help you achieve a "pump" and kick-start the muscle building process.

Glutamine

• Supplementing with Glutamine is critical to gains in strength and muscle mass. Athletes who train excessively deplete their glutamine stores. This is because they are overusing their skeletal muscles, which is where much of the glutamine in the body is stored. For more information on Glutamine, check out University of Maryland Medical Center at: www.umm.edu/altmed/articles/glutamine-000307.htm

Fat Burners

• There are many fat burners on the market that can help increase your energy, focus, suppress your appetite and may help your metabolism. My best suggestion on fat burners is to do your research of both the company and the ingredients. I also recommend consulting a Physician about possible side effects.

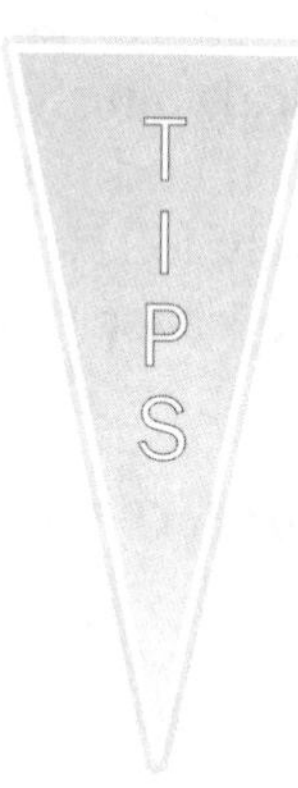

• There are 9 calories in a gram of fat.
• There are 4 calories in a gram of protein.
• There are 4 calories in a gram of carbohydrate

• Fiber is a carbohydrate but it can not be digested so when you see the term "net carbs", it refers to the carbohydrates in a food minus the fiber.

• Workout tip: training to failure is when you push your body to a point it cannot do anymore. That tells your brain it needs to adapt and become stronger.

• Workout tip: lactic acid is the burn you feel in your muscles as you fatigue them, while it is generally not liked, it is essential. The lactic acid is a key to producing growth hormone release.

Tracking Progress

I know I've said it before, but in order to be really successful on the Spike Diet©, it's important to log your daily calories. Otherwise, you are like and architect without blueprints. Many times we think we're eating less than we really are. Tracking calories allows us to see what we're eating and where we can make changes to better meet our goals. I've created a Spike Diet© Daily Food Log to help you with this. Get in the habit of having it on hand and simply jot down what you eat at each meal and snack. Another benefit to this is that you will quickly learn the nutritional information of the foods you eat; and it will become second nature. It is also helpful to keep track of your workouts using the Spike Diet© Workout Log.

Another great way to track your progress is through weekly or bi-monthly progress pictures. The pictures were the best way for me to see the results. You don't always see the small changes daily; when people would say, "Man, you've lost weight!" I could go back and look at my pictures and humbly agree. It's inspirational and gives you even more motivation to keep going.

Join an online community like the one at www.muscleandbrawn.com for support. You can also meet people with similar goals and help each other along the way. This can be a tough journey and it helps to go through it with others who can relate and keep you motivated.

Support from family, friends and community groups like the above mentioned help you achieve both your short and long-term goals. Your short-term goals will help you take it day by day and you can go to bed feeling like you've done something positive for yourself that day. Your long-term goals give you something to keep striving for. Believe me achieving your long-term goal gives you such an overwhelming feeling of empowerment. Short-term goals can be things like sticking to your calorie limit or working out for 30 minutes that day. Your long-term goal can be your ideal weight, fitting into a certain size, or competing in that triathlon you've always wanted to do. A long-term goal should be more than just a number on a scale, but a lifestyle a particular weight will allow you live, and how you feel once your there. Make sure you share your goals with your friends and family as well. They love you and want the best for you; their help and support can help you reach your full potential. When you feel overwhelmed, just relax and focus on today.

Finally, be committed and have purpose with your workouts. Intensity goes a long way when it comes to building muscle. Remember that successful diets do not starve you. You should be eating enough balanced, good quality food that you do not feel overly hungry throughout the day. You will want to stay healthy while loosing weight. And last, but certainly not least, enjoy your "Spike Day!" There is no need to feel guilty for indulging in the foods you love. Your Spike Day is an integral part of your weight loss and keeps your metabolism running strong.

The "Spike" Lifestyle

Congratulations! You have reached your goal and you should be extremely proud of your accomplishment. However, it's not over yet. Now that we are where we want to be, now is the time to be extremely cautious. We do not want to fall into our old traps and slowly bring back the habits that got us overweight in the first place.

Like I have said before, it is very important to lose weight in a way you know you can maintain. If you don't, once you go back to your regular eating habits, you will be unpleasantly surprised at how quickly each and every once returns. **Once you have reached your goal weight, you will transition to the "Spike Lifestyle."** This will ensure the weight loss is permanent.

You will no longer have a "Spike Day;" you will now have a "Spike Weekend!" I want you to begin Friday night and have a "Spike Days" through Sunday. During the week, you still need to eat good clean foods; like you did while losing weight. Also be sure to not overeat, you still have a calorie limit. However, now instead of one day, you have Friday night and two full "Spike Days" to get your cravings out. It is important to continue with your exercise routine as this is essential to overall health. Stay active and enjoy your new body!

I know from my many failed conventional diets that this is the best plan available. I can now honestly say, losing weight is not as simple as "eat less and workout more." People who say these things have no idea of what it is like to be overweight and are truly clueless to the pain and frustration of following simple diets.

On the Spike Diet©, I steamrolled to my goal weight and then easily transitioned into my new Spike Lifestyle. The weight I lost is gone for good and I never had to deprive myself of my beloved "forbidden foods."

A true key to successful dieting is commitment; the Spike Diet© is so great because it's simply 6 days of dieting and then one day to enjoy your favorite treats. This is also a guilt-free diet plan; the Spike Day is planned and important, so have fun with it. If for some reason you slip-up during the week, don't sweat it. I want you to just start again and don't look back. You are not a failure and I know you can do this. I personally "slipped" a few times before finally hitting stride the year I lost 100lbs. We are going against our own bodies design when we restrict calories to lose weight, so of course there is going to be times we are not perfect. The fact that we intentionally have a day of a calorie surplus on this diet proves to you that one "bad day" will not ruin your goals. Just push the restart button and get back on track.

I can't stress enough that it is extremely important to log your daily calories. This will show you where you are doing well and what might need refining. I have created a companion log book to help you keep track of your daily food intake and workouts. It is available on my website at: www.spikediet.com.

Always remember; on this plan you are in better shape today than you were yesterday, and tomorrow you will be in even better shape than today. So enjoy this journey. Skinny people have no idea how amazing it is to lose a lot of weight. You will have a rare opportunity to redefine yourself and become the person you have always wanted to be!

You can do this.

Russell Branjord

Author of the Spike Diet and loser of 100 pounds

SPIKE DIET© FAT-LOSS TIPS SUMMARY

- Eat more protein.
- Drink 64+ ounces of cold water each day.
- Stay away from "white death," sugar and starches.
- Have something high in protein, but low in carbohydrates, before bed.
- Do both aerobic and anaerobic (weight training) exercises.
- Cycle your calories daily with high/low days to avoid a slowdown of metabolism.
- Eat your highest calorie days on weight training days.
- Get a good amount of those calories within one hour after your workout.
- Overeating can be a habit; chew mint gum to get your mouth moving. The mint will ruin the flavor of anything you eat, and help avoid cravings.
- If you're still not satisfied, have a big glass of ice cold water.
- Avoid insulin spikes by eating protein and fiber with higher "GI" carbohydrates (see page 40).
- Eat 6-8 small meals each day to keep your metabolism high and cravings down.
- Begin each morning with a glass of ice water and whey protein. It will kick start your metabolism.
- Fat in moderation is fine; make sure you get your essential fats including
- Omega-3 and Omega-6.
- Fish oil caps and Flax Seed oil are great ways to get the "good fats."

Have a weekly Spike Day to keep your metabolism from slowing down.

THE RULES OF EFFECTIVE WORKOUTS

- Eat a balanced meal 1-2 hours before exercising.

- Have a small snack pre-workout, like a banana or apple.

- Lift weights before cardio workouts. Cardio workouts will burn the carbohydrates you need to fuel your weight lifting workout.

- Have a Whey Isolate drink immediately post workout, preferably mixed with a simple sugar like juice or Vitamin Water™. Then do your cardio workout.

- Workout with a purpose. Have intensity and focus.

- Do not over do it. It's best to split up body parts and workout for 30-45 minutes a day rather than hours at a time.

- Have a decent-sized balanced meal within an hour of working out.

- Have a slow digesting protein like eggs, milk or meat before bed.

- Get 7-8 hours of sleep a night.

- Do not work out a body part if it is still sore. Our body actually re-builds muscle while we rest; so tearing it down again before it has recovered will lead to over-training and fatigue.

FAT BURNING PRINCIPLES

- Eat less calories than you burn daily. Split your calories into several meals.
- Losing weight is as simple as calories in versus calories out.
- Fad diets are not necessary; eat a balanced diet of carbohydrates, fat and protein.
- When we diet, our brain will gradually put us in "starvation mode," much like "power-save mode" for a computer. It will slow down our metabolism so we need less energy and this is what leads to plateaus and stalled fat-loss.
- By having one day a week of a calorie surplus, you stop your declining metabolism and at the same time re-fill your muscle glycogen with glucose to fuel upcoming workouts. Eating leads to higher metabolism.
- To avoid feeling hungry, eat foods high in fiber and protein.
- It is critical to have whey protein immediately post workout. Working out will put you in a catabolic-state where your body will literally eat away at your muscles. Fueling your body with amino acids will prevent that from happening. More muscle = higher metabolism.
- Become label reader, know what you're eating and take responsibility for what you put into your body.
- Log everything; food intake, workouts, and even moods.
- The good news is that even people without great genetics and lower metabolisms can succeed and change their body composition without surgery and drugs. It just takes knowledge and discipline.

SPIKE DIET© GROCERY ESSENTIALS

- Mission Carb Balance White Flour Tortillas
- Joseph's Flax, Oat, and Wheat Pita's
- Egg Beaters or similar egg replacement
- Low fat or 2% Cheese Slices
- 2% Shredded Cheese; Mexican & Italian
- Lean ground beef or turkey
- Light hamburger Buns like Village Hearth
- Light Bread, 40-45 calories per slice
- Light English muffins like Village Hearth
- Deli meat: lean turkey, chicken and ham
- South Beach frozen entrées; pizza, etc.
- Cliff Builder or Luna bars (I like the peanut butter one)
- Beef Jerky & 2% Cheese sticks (great for snacks)
- Fiber One bars, yogurt and snacks
- Carnation Instant Breakfast (look for no sugar added)
- Balance bars and/or Nutrilite bars
- Muscle Milk and/or Nutrilite shakes
- Fresh fruit and vegetables
- Frozen vegetables – single servings
- Daisy Light sour cream
- Jimmy Dean Low fat breakfast foods
- Organic ketchup (no high fructose corn syrup)
- Canadian bacon
- Turkey hotdogs
- PB2 Powder peanut butter

SPIKE DIET© GROCERY ESSENTIALS *CONTINUED*

- Baked chips
- Quaker High Fiber Instant Oatmeal
- Pre-grilled chicken breast
- Pre-grilled chicken strips
- Coconut oil
- Center cut bacon

Note: Brands recommended are the ones that I personally have had success with. Feel free to experiment with different brands and use whichever ones you prefer.

WHERE TO FIND IT

These are the places I have found the following products. Make sure to check your local grocery stores and natural food stores as it can vary from region to region.

- Mission Carb Balance White Flour Tortillas: Cub Foods and Super Target
- Joseph's Flax, Oat and Wheat Pitas: Walmart and Cub Foods
- Nutrilite Bars and Shakes: http://tmcalpine.qhealthzone.com/
- Muscle Milk: Gas stations, Super Target, Walmart, Cub Foods and GNC
- PB2 Powdered Peanut Butter: Hy-Vee, Fitness / Nutrition shops nationwide and www.bellplantation.com
- Coconut oil: Whole Foods, Walmart, Cub Foods and Natural food stores. Coconut oil will often be found in the natural foods section of your grocery store.

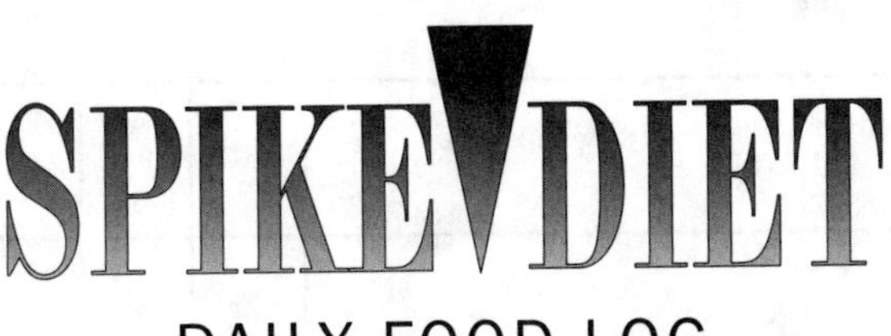

DAILY FOOD LOG

SPIKE DIET

DAILY FOOD LOG

☐ High Day ☐ Low Day

Calorie Goal 2000 Date: - -

meal	calories	protein	carbs	fiber	fat
breakfast Whey Protein Drink & *30 minutes later* Cliff Builder Bar	370	45	30	4	8
snack Apple & 2% Cheese Stick	160	6	22	5	6
lunch Subway 6-Inch Roasted Chicken on Honey Oat & Light Mayo 16 oz Skim Milk	480	39	69	5	6
snack Beef Jerky 2oz & 2% Cheese stick	230	32	4	1	7
dinner Pasta Chicken Bake w/Barilla Plus Penne & Veggies	490	44	55	9	14
snacks Low Carb Tortilla Chicken Wrap	250	21	20	11	8
TOTAL High Day= RMR Low Day = RMR - 500 Calories*	1,980	187	200	35	49

*Minimum of 1,200 Calories

Calories per Gram
Protein = 4 Calories
Carbs = 4 Calories
Fat = 9 Calories

Daily Calorie Split

- 40% Protein
- 40% Carbs
- 20% Fat
- 25+ Grams of Fiber

notes

SPIKE DIET

DAILY FOOD LOG

☐ High Day ☐ Low Day

Calorie Goal 2200 Date: - -

meal	calories	protein	carbs	fiber	fat
breakfast Whey Protein Drink, Breakfast Egg Muffin Sandwich	305	53	10	2	4.5
snack Nutrilite Energy Bar	190	14	19	0	6
lunch Burger King Plain Grilled Chicken Whopper with Ketchup	440	38	51	3	9
snack Banana pre-workout; Post-workout, Whey Protein Shake & bottle of Vitamin Water	370	41	53	0	0
dinner 2-93/7 Lean Beef Hamburgers on light buns & 2% cheese slices; side of veggie	630	63	56	12	18
snacks Low Carb Tortilla with 2 TBS of Natural Peanut Butter & 1 TBS of Chocolate Chips	348	14	40	13	21.5
TOTAL High Day= RMR Low Day = RMR - 500 Calories*	2,285	210	200	30	55

*Minimum of 1,200 Calories

Calories per Gram
Protein = 4 Calories
Carbs = 4 Calories
Fat = 9 Calories

Daily Calorie Split

- 40% Protein
- 40% Carbs
- 20% Fat
- 25+ Grams of Fiber

notes

SPIKE DIET

DAILY FOOD LOG

☐ High Day ☐ Low Day

Calorie Goal 1800 Date: - -

meal	calories	protein	carbs	fiber	fat
breakfast Strawberry Protein Smooth with Fiber One Yogurt + Strawberry Protein Powder	280	30	36	11	2
snack Nutrilite Energy Bar	190	15	19	0	6
lunch Arby's Hot Ham & Swiss Sandwich & Plain Baked Potato	470	22	81	5	8
snack Low Carb Turky Wrap	265	25	20	12	9
dinner 2-Smoked Turkey Bratwurst with light buns & side of veggies and fruit	475	33	55	11	13
snacks Nutrilite Protein Shake	160	25	4	3	6
TOTAL High Day= RMR Low Day = RMR - 500 Calories*	1,840	150	143 (28-fiber)	42	41

*Minimum of 1,200 Calories

Calories per Gram
Protein = 4 Calories
Carbs = 4 Calories
Fat = 9 Calories

Daily Calorie Split

- 40% Protein
- 40% Carbs
- 20% Fat
- 25+ Grams of Fiber

notes

SPIKE DIET

DAILY FOOD LOG

☐ High Day ☐ Low Day

Calorie Goal 1200 Date: - -

meal	calories	protein	carbs	fiber	fat
breakfast Carnation Instant Breakfast, No Sugar Added Ready-to-Drink Shake; Water with pure fiber powder	190	13	25	11	5
snack Balance Bar	200	14	23	1	6
lunch Turkey Hotdog, Light bun & ketchup 1/2 serving baked lays	200	12	30	3	4
snack Fiber One Bar	140	4	29	9	4
dinner Grilled Chicken Breast with 2% shredded Mozzarella Cheese & 1/4 cup pizza or tomato sauce	225	29	6	0	9
snacks Cliff Builder Bar	270	20	30	4	8
TOTAL High Day= RMR Low Day = RMR - 500 Calories*	1,225	92	143 (28-fiber)	28	36

*Minimum of 1,200 Calories

Calories per Gram
Protein = 4 Calories
Carbs = 4 Calories
Fat = 9 Calories

Daily Calorie Split

- 40% Protein
- 40% Carbs
- 20% Fat
- 25+ Grams of Fiber

notes

SPIKE DIET

DAILY FOOD LOG

☐ High Day ☐ Low Day

Calorie Goal 1500 Date: - -

meal	calories	protein	carbs	fiber	fat
breakfast 2-Kashi Waffles with sugar free syrup & 2 turkey sausage links	290	21	34	6	10
snack Cliff Builder Bar	270	20	30	4	8
lunch Low Carb Turkey Wrap, 2% sliced cheese & 1 TBS fat free mayo/sour cream	265	25	20	12	6
snack Apple & Post Workout Whey Shake 1 scoop with water	160	25	20	4	0
dinner Ground turkey soft taco 2% cheese & mission low carb wrap with light sour cream	365	36	20	12	15
snacks beef/turkey jerky & 2% cheese stick	170	23	3	0	7
TOTAL High Day= RMR Low Day = RMR - 500 Calories*	1,520	145	126 (38-fiber)	38	46

*Minimum of 1,200 Calories

Calories per Gram
Protein = 4 Calories
Carbs = 4 Calories
Fat = 9 Calories

Daily Calorie Split

- 40% Protein
- 40% Carbs
- 20% Fat
- 25+ Grams of Fiber

notes

SPIKE DIET

DAILY FOOD LOG

☐ High Day ☐ Low Day

Calorie Goal 1500 Date: - -

meal	calories	protein	carbs	fiber	fat
breakfast 2-Kashi Waffles with sugar free syrup & 2 turkey sausage links	290	21	34	6	10
snack Nutralite Meal Bar	180	14	26	4	8
lunch Low Carb Turkey Wrap, 2% sliced cheese & 1 TBS fat free mayo/sour cream	265	25	20	12	6
snack Apple & Post Workout Whey Shake 1 scoop with water	160	25	20	4	0
dinner Ground turkey soft taco 2% cheese & mission low carb wrap with light sour cream	365	36	20	12	15
snacks beef/turkey jerky & 2% cheese stick	170	23	3	0	7
TOTAL High Day= RMR Low Day = RMR - 500 Calories*	1,480	139	122 (38-fiber)	38	46

*Minimum of 1,200 Calories

Calories per Gram
Protein = 4 Calories
Carbs = 4 Calories
Fat = 9 Calories

Daily Calorie Split

- 40% Protein
- 40% Carbs
- 20% Fat
- 25+ Grams of Fiber

notes

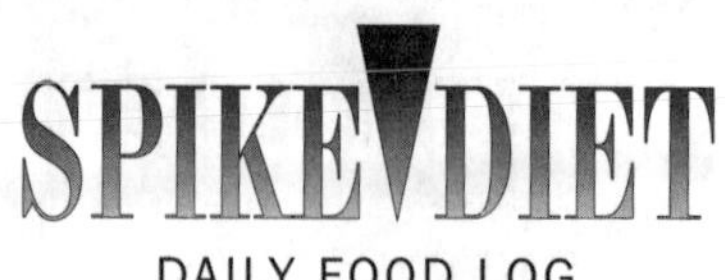

DAILY FOOD LOG

☐ High Day ☐ Low Day

Calorie Goal 1500 Date: - -

meal	calories	protein	carbs	fiber	fat
breakfast 3-oatmeal pancakes with 2 slices of Canadian Bacon	358	18	69	8	4.5
snack Nutralite Protein Shake RTD	170	25	6	4	6
lunch Healthy Choice Soup and apple pre-workout	240	12	48	8	3
snack Post Workout Whey Shake 1 sccop with water and banana	160	25	27	1	0
dinner Fiesta Lime Chicken with 2% cheese and lime juice 2 tortilla chips crushed on top	250	37	4	0	9
snacks low carb tortilla with 1 TBS peanut butter	298	13	25	13	19
TOTAL High Day= RMR Low Day = RMR - 500 Calories*	1,526	131	178 (33-fiber)	33	41

*Minimum of 1,200 Calories

Calories per Gram
Protein = 4 Calories
Carbs = 4 Calories
Fat = 9 Calories

Daily Calorie Split

- 40% Protein
- 40% Carbs
- 20% Fat
- 25+ Grams of Fiber

notes

SPIKE DIET

DAILY FOOD LOG

☐ High Day ☐ Low Day

Calorie Goal 1500 Date: - -

meal	calories	protein	carbs	fiber	fat
breakfast 3-oatmeal pancakes with 2 slices of Canadian Bacon	358	18	69	8	4.5
snack Nutralite Protein Shake RTD	170	25	6	4	6
lunch Healthy Choice Soup and apple pre-workout	240	12	48	8	3
snack Post Workout Whey Shake 1 sccop with water and banana	160	25	27	1	0
dinner Fiesta Lime Chicken with 2% cheese and lime juice 2 tortilla chips crushed on top	250	37	4	0	9
snacks low carb tortilla with 1 TBS peanut butter	298	13	25	13	19
TOTAL High Day= RMR Low Day = RMR - 500 Calories*	1,526	131	178 (33-fiber)	33	41

*Minimum of 1,200 Calories

Calories per Gram
Protein = 4 Calories
Carbs = 4 Calories
Fat = 9 Calories

Daily Calorie Split

- 40% Protein
- 40% Carbs
- 20% Fat
- 25+ Grams of Fiber

notes

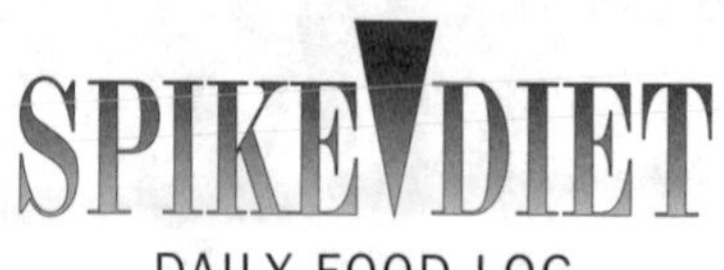

DAILY FOOD LOG

☐ High Day ☐ Low Day

Calorie Goal 1500 Date: - -

meal	calories	protein	carbs	fiber	fat
breakfast Whey Protein Drink & 30 minutes later, Open Face Egg Muffin with 2% cheese & Canadian Bacon, cup of strawberries	382	54	30	7	4.5
snack Nutrilite Chocolate Nut Roll Energy Bar	190	15	19	0	6
lunch Turkey & Cheese Sandwich and Apple, pre-workout	245	22	41	8	3
snack Post Workout Whey Shake 1 scoop with water & Vitamin Water	180	25	18	0	0
dinner Shredded Barbeque Chicken Sandwich on Village Hearth Light Bun & side of veggies	290	18	39	7	3.5
snacks Cliff Builder Bar	270	20	30	4	8
TOTAL High Day= RMR Low Day = RMR - 500 Calories*	1,557	154	177 (26-fiber)	26	25

*Minimum of 1,200 Calories

Calories per Gram
Protein = 4 Calories
Carbs = 4 Calories
Fat = 9 Calories

Daily Calorie Split

- 40% Protein
- 40% Carbs
- 20% Fat
- 25+ Grams of Fiber

notes

SPIKE DIET

DAILY FOOD LOG

☐ High Day ☐ Low Day

Calorie Goal 1200 Date: - -

meal	calories	protein	carbs	fiber	fat
breakfast Jimmy Dean De-Light Breakfast Sandwich	260	18	30	2	7
snack Carnation Instant Breakfast RTD no sugar added	140	13	14	2	5
lunch Hot Roast Beef & Cheese Sandwich on Village Hearth Light Bun	245	28	18	3	7.5
snack Nutrilite Protein Shake	170	25	6	4	6
dinner Grilled Fajita Chicken on Low Carb Tortilla & Veggies	210	27	22	13	3.5
snacks High Fiber and Protein Pizza	235	27	16	8	8
TOTAL High Day= RMR Low Day = RMR - 500 Calories*	1,260	138	106	32	37

*Minimum of 1,200 Calories

Daily Calorie Split

- 40% Protein
- 40% Carbs
- 20% Fat
- 25+ Grams of Fiber

Calories per Gram
Protein = 4 Calories
Carbs = 4 Calories
Fat = 9 Calories

notes

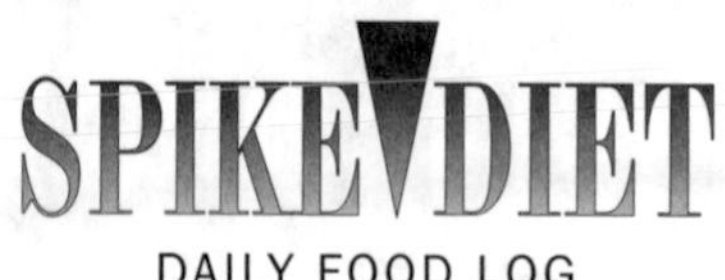

DAILY FOOD LOG

☐ High Day ☐ Low Day

Calorie Goal 1400 Date: - -

meal	calories	protein	carbs	fiber	fat
breakfast 1 cup high fiber cereal such as Fiber One Honey Clusters with 1 cup skim milk	240	1.5	53	13	13
snack low-fat string cheese with 1 serving Baked Lays	200	6	25	1	10
lunch Breakfast Burrito w/ salsa	215	21	22	11	6
snack Slice of Oatmeal Bran Cake & Fiber One Yogurt	210	7	48	9	2
dinner Greek Turkey Burgers side of veggies	310	35	18	5	9
snacks Canadian Bacon Pizza	235	27	16	8	8
TOTAL High Day= RMR Low Day = RMR - 500 Calories*	1,420	97	182	47	48

*Minimum of 1,200 Calories

Calories per Gram
Protein = 4 Calories
Carbs = 4 Calories
Fat = 9 Calories

Daily Calorie Split

- 40% Protein
- 40% Carbs
- 20% Fat
- 25+ Grams of Fiber

notes

SPIKE DIET

DAILY FOOD LOG

☐ High Day ☐ Low Day

Calorie Goal 1300 Date: - -

meal	calories	protein	carbs	fiber	fat
breakfast Balance Bar	200	15	23	1	6
snack High Fiber Peanut Butter Yogurt Salad	180	7	29	11	3
lunch 1 serving of a Healthy Choice Soup with an apple	190	8	33	7	1
snack Banana	115	1	27	3	0
dinner Taco Salad	290	23	25	7	10
snacks South Beach Pizza	350	31	36	9	12
TOTAL High Day= RMR Low Day = RMR - 500 Calories*	1325	85	173	38	32

*Minimum of 1,200 Calories

Calories per Gram
Protein = 4 Calories
Carbs = 4 Calories
Fat = 9 Calories

Daily Calorie Split

- 40% Protein
- 40% Carbs
- 20% Fat
- 25+ Grams of Fiber

notes

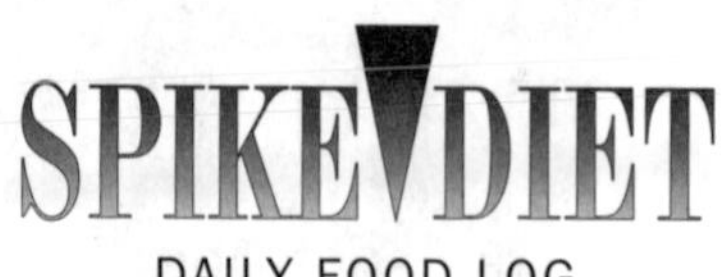

DAILY FOOD LOG

☐ High Day ☐ Low Day

Calorie Goal 1900 Date: - -

meal	calories	protein	carbs	fiber	fat
breakfast Breakfast Burrito, 8 ounces skim milk	295	29	33	11	6
snack 1/2 cup cottage cheese mixed with 1/8 cup sunflower seeds and a few sliced green olives	180	16	7	4	8
lunch South Beach Pizza, 8 ounces skim milk, carrot sticks	430	39	47	9	12
snack 1 medium apple, sliced 2 TBS peanut butter	260	8	25	5	16
dinner Turkey Burger on a light bun, slice of 2% cheese, 2 strips center cut baon sweet potato fries	495	39	41	6	20
snacks Cliff Bar	270	20	33	4	8
TOTAL High Day= RMR Low Day = RMR - 500 Calories*	1930	151	186	39	70

*Minimum of 1,200 Calories

Calories per Gram
Protein = 4 Calories
Carbs = 4 Calories
Fat = 9 Calories

Daily Calorie Split

- 40% Protein
- 40% Carbs
- 20% Fat
- 25+ Grams of Fiber

notes

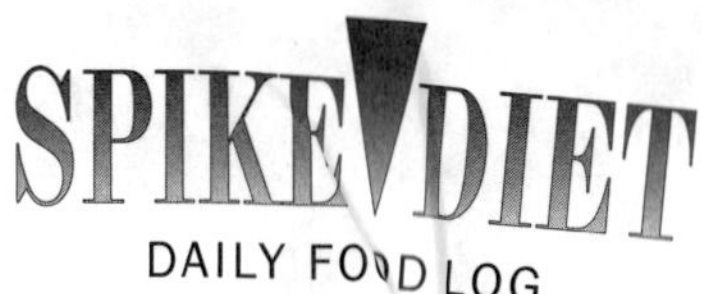

☐ High Day ☐ Low Day

Calorie Goal 1200 | e: - -

meal	calories	protein	carbs	r	fat
breakfast 1/2 light English muffin & 1/2 cup Egg Beater's Cheese and Chive	120	12	11	2	4
snack Cliff Bar	270	20	30	4	8
lunch Chicken Bacon Ranch Pizza	185	23	9	4	
snack Carrot Sticks w/2 tbsp light ranch	105	2	11	2	7
dinner Chicken CousCous w/carrots	190	20	18	0	2
snacks South Beach Pizza	350	31	33	9	12
TOTAL High Day= RMR Low Day = RMR - 500 Calories*	1220	108	112	21	40

*Minimum of 1,200 Calories

Daily Calorie Split

- 40% Protein
- 40% Carbs
- 20% Fat
- 25+ Grams of Fiber

Calories per Gram
Protein = 4 Calories
Carbs = 4 Calories
Fat = 9 Calories

notes

SPIKE DIET

DAILY FOOD LOG

☐ High Day ☐ Low Day

Calorie Goal 1200 Date: - -

meal	calories	protein	carbs	fiber	fat
breakfast Cliff Ba	120	12	11	2	4
snack Carro cks with 2 TBS light ranch dressing	270	20	30	4	8
lunch en muffin pizza 8 es skim milk	185	23	9	4	7
of Oatmeal Bran Cake	105	2	11	2	7
r e Pan Tacos	190	20	18	0	2
acks 5 slices of turkey pepperoni with 1/4 cup shredded 2% cheese to make "pepperoni tacos"	350	31	33	9	12
TOTAL High Day= RMR Low Day = RMR - 500 Calories*	1220	108	112	21	40

*Minimum of 1,200 Calories

Calories per Gram
Protein = 4 Calories
Carbs = 4 Calories
Fat = 9 Calories

Daily Calorie Split

- 40% Protein
- 40% Carbs
- 20% Fat
- 25+ Grams of Fiber

notes

SPIKE DIET

DAILY FOOD LOG

☐ High Day ☐ Low Day

Calorie Goal 1400 Date: - -

meal	calories	protein	carbs	fiber	fat
breakfast Egg Mess	320	34	35	4	5
snack Fiber One Bar	140	2	29	9	4
lunch Southwestern BLT Wraps 1 serving tortilla chips with salsa	335	15	55	15	7
snack Fiber One Yogurt with flaxseed	140	6	17	8	6
dinner Turkey Picadillo	270	27	34	7	3
snacks Chicken Bacon Ranch Pizza	185	23	9	4	7
TOTAL High Day= RMR Low Day = RMR - 500 Calories*	1390	107	179	47	42

*Minimum of 1,200 Calories

Daily Calorie Split

- 40% Protein
- 40% Carbs
- 20% Fat
- 25+ Grams of Fiber

Calories per Gram
Protein = 4 Calories
Carbs = 4 Calories
Fat = 9 Calories

notes

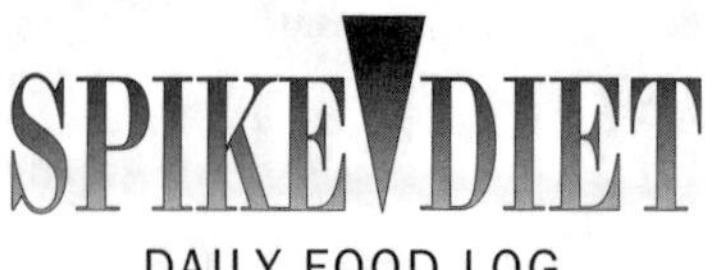

DAILY FOOD LOG

☐ High Day ☐ Low Day

Calorie Goal 1400 Date: - -

meal	calories	protein	carbs	fiber	fat
breakfast High Fiber Apple Cinnamon Oatmeal	232	8	58	15	2
snack Low-Carb Tortilla Strips with 2 TBS hummus	200	8	26	13	8
lunch Summer Salad with Chicken 1 serving Baked Lays	305	17	40	3	9
snack HIgh FIber Peanut Butter Yogurt Salad	180	7	29	11	3
dinner Chicken and Cheese Tortellini Soup with slice of light toast	255	25	34	4	4
snacks Fiber One Bar	200	15	23	0	6
TOTAL High Day= RMR Low Day = RMR - 500 Calories*	1372	80	210	46	32

*Minimum of 1,200 Calories

Calories per Gram
Protein = 4 Calories
Carbs = 4 Calories
Fat = 9 Calories

Daily Calorie Split

- 40% Protein
- 40% Carbs
- 20% Fat
- 25+ Grams of Fiber

notes

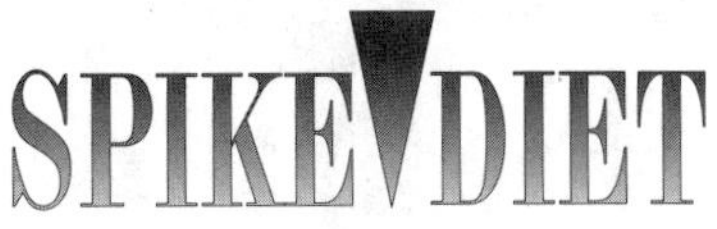

DAILY FOOD LOG

☐ High Day ☐ Low Day

Calorie Goal 1400 Date: - -

meal	calories	protein	carbs	fiber	fat
breakfast High Fiber Cottage	175	15	23	4	2
snack Apple with 2 TBS peanut butter	260	8	25	5	16
lunch South Beach Pizza	350	31	33	9	12
snack low-carb tortilla strips w/hummus	155	7	24	13	3
dinner Chicken Stir Fry	273	28	32	4	2
snacks Luna Bar	180	9	26	3	5
TOTAL High Day= RMR Low Day = RMR - 500 Calories*	1393	98	163	38	40

*Minimum of 1,200 Calories

Calories per Gram
Protein = 4 Calories
Carbs = 4 Calories
Fat = 9 Calories

Daily Calorie Split

- 40% Protein
- 40% Carbs
- 20% Fat
- 25+ Grams of Fiber

notes

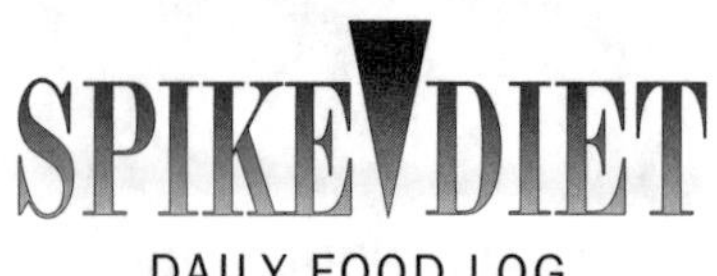

DAILY FOOD LOG

☐ High Day ☐ Low Day

Calorie Goal 1200 Date: - -

meal	calories	protein	carbs	fiber	fat
breakfast 1/2 light English muffin 1/2 cup Egg Beater's scrambled	120	12	11	2	4
snack Cliff Bar	270	20	30	4	8
lunch Chicken Bacon Ranch Pizza	185	23	9	4	7
snack Carrot Sticks with 1 TBS light ranch	105	2	11	2	7
dinner Chicken CousCous with carrots	190	20	18	0	2
snacks South Beach Pizza	350	31	33	9	12
TOTAL High Day= RMR Low Day = RMR - 500 Calories*	1220	108	112	21	40

*Minimum of 1,200 Calories

Calories per Gram
Protein = 4 Calories
Carbs = 4 Calories
Fat = 9 Calories

Daily Calorie Split

- 40% Protein
- 40% Carbs
- 20% Fat
- 25+ Grams of Fiber

notes

SPIKE DIET

DAILY FOOD LOG

☐ High Day ☐ Low Day

Calorie Goal 1500 Date: - -

meal	calories	protein	carbs	fiber	fat
breakfast Low-fat french toast with Fiber One Yogurt	315	22	58	13	2
snack Handful of almonds	165	5	7	3	13
lunch Sliders	350	25	48	6	8
snack Banana	105	1	26	3	0
dinner Beef Chilaquiles	390	37	25	2	19
snacks NO-Bake Chewy Protein Bar	190	16	23	5	4
TOTAL High Day= RMR Low Day = RMR - 500 Calories*	1515	106	187	32	46

*Minimum of 1,200 Calories

Calories per Gram
Protein = 4 Calories
Carbs = 4 Calories
Fat = 9 Calories

Daily Calorie Split

- 40% Protein
- 40% Carbs
- 20% Fat
- 25+ Grams of Fiber

notes

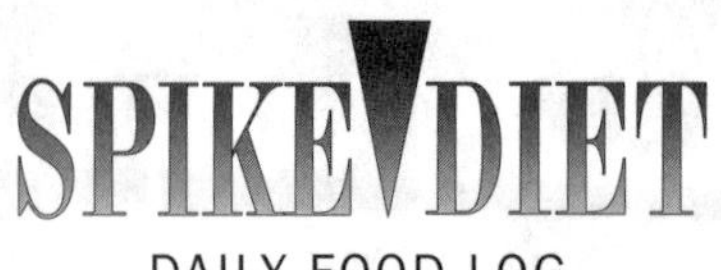

DAILY FOOD LOG

☐ High Day ☐ Low Day

Calorie Goal 2300 Date: - -

meal	calories	protein	carbs	fiber	fat
breakfast 2-Oatmeal Waffles w/sugar free syrup	400	10	62	8	20
snack Breakfast Salad	375	12	71	8	7
lunch Chicken and Cheese Quesadilla w/2-Carb Balance Tortillas	524	47	42	22	13
snack 14 oz Muscle Milk	230	25	12	2	9
dinner Chicken Pasta Bake	495	44	47	5	14
snacks Cliff Bar	270	20	30	4	8
TOTAL High Day= RMR Low Day = RMR - 500 Calories*	2294	158	264	49	45

*Minimum of 1,200 Calories

Daily Calorie Split

- 40% Protein
- 40% Carbs
- 20% Fat
- 25+ Grams of Fiber

Calories per Gram
Protein = 4 Calories
Carbs = 4 Calories
Fat = 9 Calories

notes

SPIKE DIET

DAILY FOOD LOG

☐ High Day ☐ Low Day

Calorie Goal 1200 Date: - -

meal	calories	protein	carbs	fiber	fat
breakfast Open Face Egg Muffin	205	28	10	2	4.5
snack 3 cups air popped popcorn	170	12	30	2	3
lunch Turkey, Apple and Swiss Sandwich	240	29	27	5	2
snack Low-Carb Tortilla Strips with salsa	145	7	23	13	3
dinner Mini Veggie Pizzas	210	16	20	7	7
snacks Balance Bar	270	20	30	4	8
TOTAL High Day= RMR Low Day = RMR - 500 Calories*	1240	112	140	35	27

*Minimum of 1,200 Calories

Calories per Gram
Protein = 4 Calories
Carbs = 4 Calories
Fat = 9 Calories

Daily Calorie Split

- 40% Protein
- 40% Carbs
- 20% Fat
- 25+ Grams of Fiber

notes

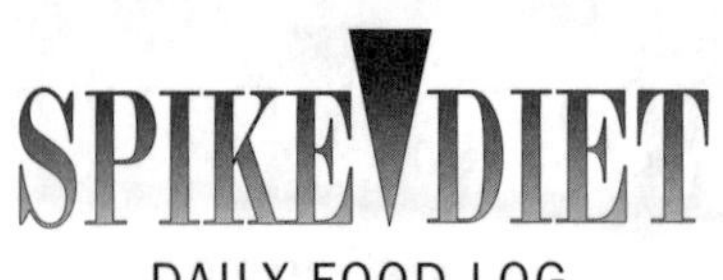

DAILY FOOD LOG

☐ High Day ☐ Low Day

Calorie Goal 1600 Date: - -

meal	calories	protein	carbs	fiber	fat
breakfast Peanut Butter Banana Smoothie	415	24	72	8	4
snack 2% or Low-Fat String Cheese 1 serving Baked Chips	190	9	24	1	6
lunch Healthy Choice Pasta Bowl	340	15	56	8	6
snack 1/2 cup cottage cheese with one pear	175	15	21	4	2
dinner Egg and Cheese Stuffing Bake	226	22	15	1	7
snacks Canadian Bacon Pizza	235	27	16	8	8
TOTAL High Day= RMR Low Day = RMR - 500 Calories*	1581	112	204	30	33

*Minimum of 1,200 Calories

Calories per Gram
Protein = 4 Calories
Carbs = 4 Calories
Fat = 9 Calories

Daily Calorie Split

- 40% Protein
- 40% Carbs
- 20% Fat
- 25+ Grams of Fiber

notes

SPIKE DIET

DAILY FOOD LOG

☐ High Day ☐ Low Day

Calorie Goal 1300	Date: - -

meal	calories	protein	carbs	fiber	fat
breakfast Sandra's High Fiber Smoothie	170	12	34	7	0
snack Tortilla Roll-Ups	260	23	20	11	8
lunch Bacon Grilled Cheese, 1/4 cup grapes 1 serving Baked Lays	365	20	48	4	8
snack Fresh veggies with Light Ranch Dressing	140	3	23	5	7
dinner Sloppy Jose's	210	17	24	4	5
snacks Balance Bar	200	15	23	0	6
TOTAL High Day= RMR Low Day = RMR - 500 Calories*	1345	90	172	31	34

*Minimum of 1,200 Calories

Calories per Gram
Protein = 4 Calories
Carbs = 4 Calories
Fat = 9 Calories

Daily Calorie Split

- 40% Protein
- 40% Carbs
- 20% Fat
- 25+ Grams of Fiber

notes

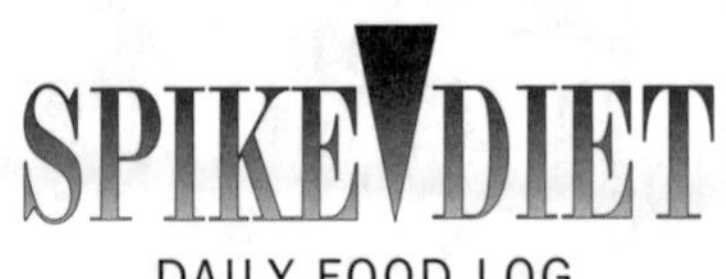

DAILY FOOD LOG

☐ High Day ☐ Low Day

Calorie Goal 1300 Date: - -

meal	calories	protein	carbs	fiber	fat
breakfast 2 slices light toast with 1 TBS peanut butter each slice, 1/2 cup strawberries	170	12	34	7	0
snack 1 serving Baked Tostitos with salsa	260	23	20	11	8
lunch A frozen veggies for One with 1 grilled chicken breast	365	20	48	4	8
snack Fiber One Bar	140	3	23	5	7
dinner Bean and Cheese Quesadillas 1 serving Mexicorn	210	17	24	4	5
snacks English Muffin Pizza	200	15	23	0	6
TOTAL High Day= RMR Low Day = RMR - 500 Calories*	1345	90	172	31	34

*Minimum of 1,200 Calories

Calories per Gram
Protein = 4 Calories
Carbs = 4 Calories
Fat = 9 Calories

Daily Calorie Split

- 40% Protein
- 40% Carbs
- 20% Fat
- 25+ Grams of Fiber

notes

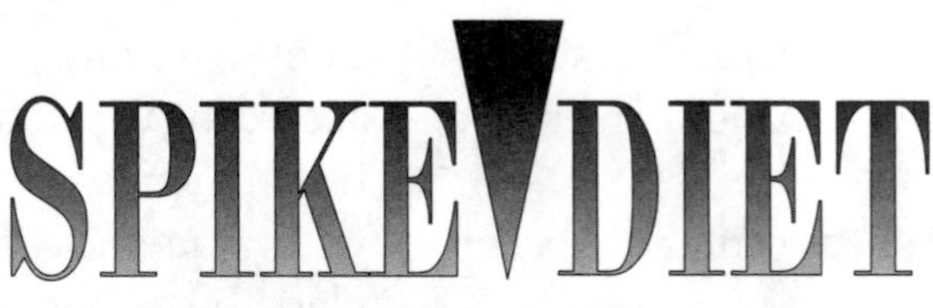

APPROVED RECIPES

Bacon & Turkey Grilled Cheese

2 slices light Italian Bread

1 slice Kraft 2% singles American cheese

2 slices center cut bacon

2 slices smoked deli turkey

Non-stick cooking spray

INSTRUCTIONS

Cook bacon in microwave according to package directions. Lightly spray one slice of bread with non-stick cooking spray, place on a non-stick pan over med-high heat. Top with one slice of cheese, turkey and bacon. Lightly spray the other piece of bread and place on top. Cook until lightly browned, flip and cook the other side until lightly browned. These are good for a quick lunch.

NUTRTION INFO

Makes 1 serving
(One Large Serving)

205 calories
6 grams of fat
18 grams of carbs
3 grams of fiber
18 grams of protein

BBQ Chicken Sandwiches

5 oz Boneless Skinless Chicken Breast

2 Tbsp Barbecue Sauce

2 slices Light Sliced Cheese

2 Light Wheat Hamburger Buns

INSTRUCTIONS

Place raw chicken breast in a pot with cold water; cook over medium heat for approximately 20 minutes until chicken is cooked through. Rinse chicken under cold water and shred with two forks. Add barbecue sauce to shredded chicken and mix to coat. Place half of the chicken on one bun, top with cheese. Repeat for second sandwich.

Tasty tip: Before adding the chicken, spritz the buns with a touch of butter PAM. Place in the oven and broil on each side for a couple of minutes.

From Lorin Elise

NUTRTION INFO

Makes 1 serving (2 sandwiches)
(Two Sandwiches)

500 calories
13 grams of fat
55 grams of carbs
4.5 grams of fiber
48 grams of protein

Beef Chilaquiles

93/7 Ground Beef or Turkey

1 Mission Low-Carb Tortilla

½ cup Egg Beaters

1/4 cup 2% shredded cheese, Mexican or Colby Jack

1/4 cup salsa

Baked Tostitos and Daisy Light Sour Cream

INSTRUCTIONS

Heat oven to 350. Brown meat in a large skillet. Stir in enchilada sauce. Sprinkle have of the crushed Tostitos on the bottom of a 2 qt baking dish and top with half the ground meat mixture and half of the 2% shredded cheese. Layer once more; chips, meat, cheese. Bake for 15 minutes. Top with lettuce or diced tomatoes if desired and up to 2 Tbl of Daisy Light Sour Cream.

NUTRTION INFO

Makes 4 servings
(One Large Serving)

390 calories
19 grams of fat
25 grams of carbs
2 grams of fiber
37 grams of protein

Breakfast Salad

1/4 cup old fashioned oatmeal

1/2 apple, cut up

1 banana, sliced

1 Tbsp chopped walnuts

1/2 Tbsp ground flaxseed

1 container vanilla Fiber One yogurt

INSTRUCTIONS:

Mix together oats, apple, banana, and walnuts. Top with yogurt and flaxseed.

NUTRTION INFO

Makes 1 Serving
(One Large Serving)

375 calories
7 grams of fat
71 grams of carbs
8 grams of fiber
12 grams of protein

Canadian Bacon Pizza

2-Josepth Flax, Oat, Whole Wheat Pita Bread (Thank's Andy) found at Cub Foods

1/4 Cup of 2% Mozzarella Cheese

3 Slices of Canadian Bacon

1/4 Cup of Pizza Sauce

INSTRUCTIONS

Heat oven to 350. Cut Canadian Bacon slices into 8 pieces. Top pitas with pizza sauce, cheese and Canadian Bacon. Bake for 8 minutes. These get rave reviews and are another favorite bedtime snack of mine.

NUTRTION INFO

(2 Full Pita Rounds)

235 calories
8 grams of fat
16 grams of carbs
8 grams of fiber
27 grams of protein

Chewy No-Bake Protein Bars

2 cups rolled oats

1 1/2 cups chocolate whey protein powder

1 Tbsp cinnamon

2 tsp vanilla

1/4 cup honey

1/2 cup PB2

1/4 cup water

INSTRUCTIONS

Mix PB2 with water as per package instructions. In a small bowl, stir together oats, protein powder and cinnamon. Set aside. In a medium microwave safe bowl, combine vanilla, honey PB2 and water. Microwave at 20 second intervals until ingredients are well mixed. Add oat mixture little by little and mix as well as possible-this part may take awhile as the mixture is hard to stir. Spread in a baking pan and place in refrigerator to harden. Cut into 8 bars. Wrap each individually in wax paper and store in fridge.

NUTRTION INFO

Makes 8 Servings

(One Serving)

190 calories

4 grams of fat

23 grams of carbs

5 grams of fiber

16 grams of protein

Chicken and Tortellini Soup

3 cups reduced-fat low sodium chicken broth

3 cups water

1/2 tsp Italian seasoning

1 9oz package of refrigerated cheese tortellini

1 package of precooked, diced chicken chunks

3 carrots, peeled and thinly sliced

4 plum tomatoes, chopped

1 6oz bag of baby spinach

INSTRUCTIONS

Bring broth, water, and seasoning to boil in a large pot. Pour in the tortellini and reduce heat to med-low, simmer for 3 minutes. Add carrots and simmer for 4 minutes, then stir in the baby spinach and tomatoes and simmer for 2 minutes or until carrots are tender.

NUTRTION INFO

Makes 4 servings
(One Large Serving)

215 calories
4 grams of fat
25 grams of carbs
3 grams of fiber
22 grams of protein

Chicken Bacon Ranch Pizza

2 Joseph's Pitas

1/4 cup 2% shredded mozzerella cheese

3 slices center cut bacon

3 oz pre-cooked chicken strips

1 Tbl light Ranch dressing

INSTRUCTIONS

Heat oven to 350. Cook bacon in microwave according to package instructions. Spread Ranch dressing in a thin layer, dividing evenly among the 2 pitas. Top with chicken strips, cheese, and bacon. Bake in oven for 8 minutes. This is one of my favorite before bed snacks-very delicious!

NUTRTION INFO

Makes 2 Servings

(One Serving)

185 calories

7 grams of fat

9 grams of carbs

4 grams of fiber

23 grams protien

Chicken Couscous with Carrots

1 lb cooked chicken breasts, cut into chunks

2 cups reduced-fat chicken broth

1/2 tsp cumin

1/2 tsp ground cinnamon

1/2 cup shredded carrots or 2 carrots peeled and thinly sliced

1 tomato, chopped

1 cup plain couscous

INSTRUCTIONS

Pour chicken broth in large skillet, add cumin, cinnamon and carrots. Cover and simmer for 10 minutes or until tender. Meanwhile, microwave chicken chunks until warm. Remove broth mixture from the heat and stir in the tomatoes, chicken and couscous. Cover for 5 minutes, then fluff with a fork. Season with salt and pepper if desired.

NUTRTION INFO

Makes 4 servings

(One Large Serving)

190 calories

2 grams of fat

18 grams of carbs

3 grams of fiber

20 grams of protein

Chicken Enchiladas

2 cans enchilada sauce

2 cups cooked chicken, cut up in chunks

1 cup black beans, drained and rinsed

1 package taco seasoning mix

8 low-carb tortillas

1 cup 2% shredded Mexican cheese

INSTRUCTIONS

Heat oven to 350. Spray a 9 x 13 baking dish with cooking spray and pour 1/2 can of enchilada sauce over the bottom. Mix together chicken, 1 can enchilada sauce, black beans and taco seasoning. Heat in a non-stick skillet over medium until heated through. Divide chicken mixture evenly among tortillas, roll-up, and place seam side down in baking dish. Top with remaining ½ can enchilada sauce and shredded cheese. Bake 20 minutes or until hot.

NUTRTION INFO

Makes 8 Enchiladas

(One Enchilada)

265 calories

6 grams of fat

25 grams of carbs

13 grams of fiber

27 grams of protein

Chicken Parmesean

4 Boneless Skinless Chicken Breasts

1 14 oz Jar of Pasta Sauce

1 cup Shredded 2% Mozzerella Cheese

1/2 a box of Barilla Plus Penne Pasta

INSTRUCTIONS

Heat oven to 375. Pour ½ of the sauce on the bottom of a 9x12 baking dish. Top with chicken and pour the rest of the sauce over the chicken. Cover with foil and bake for 30 minutes. Uncover, sprinkle with 2% shredded mozzarella cheese and bake 5 minutes or until chicken is done. Serve over Barilla Plus pasta.

NUTRTION INFO

Makes 4 servings
(One Large Serving)

490 calories
10 grams of fat
57 grams of carbs
7 grams of fiber
44 grams of protein

Chicken Pasta Bake

1/2 Cup of Barilla Plus Penne

3 oz of Grilled Chicken cubed

1/2 Cup of Shredded 2% Mozzarella Cheese

1/4 Cup of pasta sauce

INSTRUCTIONS

Boil pasta and warm chicken in microwave, I use Tyson pre-grilled chicken breast strips.

Mix sauce and chicken into the pasta, add place microwave safe plate and top with cheese

Microwave for 20-30 seconds until cheese has melted.

NUTRTION INFO

(One Large Serving)

495 calories

14 grams of fat

47 grams of carbs

5 grams of fiber

44 grams of protein

Chicken Ranch Wraps

3 oz ready to eat grilled chicken strips

2 Mission low-carb tortillas

2 Tbsp fat-free Ranch dressing

1/2 cup 2% shredded Colby Jack Cheese

Shredded lettuce

INSTRUCTIONS

Spread 1 Tbsp of fat-free Ranch dressing on each low-carb tortilla. Divide chicken and cheese evenly among tortillas, top with shredded lettuce and roll up.

NUTRTION INFO

Makes 1 serving (One Wrap)

241 calories
8 grams of fat
23 grams of carbs
11 grams of fiber
22 grams of protein

Chicken Stir Fry

1lb boneless skinless chicken breasts, cut into strips

1/4 cup fat-free Italian dressing

1 Tbsp soy sauce

1/2 tsp minced garlic

1 red pepper, chopped

1 cup baby carrots

1 cup snap peas

3 servings brown rice, cooked

INSTRUCTIONS

Mix fat-free Italian dressing, soy sauce and garlic together. Add 1 Tbsp of the sauce to the chicken and coat, let stand for 5 minutes. Heat 1 Tbsp Canola oil in a large wok or non-stick skillet over med-high heat. Add meat and vegetables and stir-fry for 4 minutes or until meat is done. Pour the rest of the dressing mix over and simmer for 1 minute. Serve over brown rice.

NUTRTION INFO

Makes 4 servings

(One Large Serving)

273 calories

2 grams of fat

31 grams of carbs

4 grams of fiber

28 grams of protein

Cream Cheese Turkey Tortilla Wraps

1 low-carb tortilla

3 slices deli turkey

2 Tbsp 1/3 less fat cream cheese

1/4 cup shredded
2% cheddar cheese

Dill pickles-optional

INSTRUCTIONS

Spread cream cheese on tortilla. Sprinkle shredded cheese and top with turkey and sliced pickles if desired, roll up.

I like to make several of these and then slice them up into finger food snacks and keep them individual wrapped in zip lock bags for quick convenient snacks!

NUTRTION INFO

Makes 1 serving
(One Large Serving)

260 calories
8 grams of fat
20 grams of carbs
11 grams of fiber
23 grams of protein

English Muffin Egg Sandwich

1/2 Cup Egg Beater

1/2 Light English Muffin

Slice of 2% Cheese

3 Slices of Canadian Bacon

INSTRUCTIONS

Toast one half of light english muffin, Cook egg beaters on lightly sprayed skillet. Warm 3 Slices of Canadian Bacon in Microwave

Top English Muffin with eggs, canadian bacon & 2% sliced Cheese

Warm in microwave about 10 seconds until cheese is melted.

NUTRTION INFO

Makes 1 Serving
(1/2 Muffin and toppins)

205 calories
4.5 grams of fat
10 grams of carbs
2 grams of fiber
28 grams of protein

Egg and Cheese Stuffing Bake

1 ¼ cups Egg Beaters

1 cup Skim Milk

1/2 cup Daisy Light Sour Cream

1 small zucchini, sliced

2 cups stuffing mix, unprepared

2 Turkey Hot Dogs or Fat Free Beef Hot Dogs, cut into chunks

1 cup shredded 2% Colby Jack Cheese

INSTRUCTIONS

Heat oven to 375. Mix together Egg Beaters, milk and sour cream by hand. Stir in zucchini, stuffing, hot dogs and ½ cup cheese until just mixed. Pour into a 9-inch pie plate and cover loosely with foil. Bake for 1 hour, uncover, top with remaining cheese and bake for 5 additional minutes.

NUTRTION INFO

Makes 5 servings
(One Large Serving)

226 calories
7 grams of fat
15 grams of carbs
1 gram of fiber
22 grams of protein

English Muffin Pizzas

1 english muffin, split

2 tbsp pizza sauce

1/4 cup shredded mozzerella cheese

6 slices turkey pepperoni

INSTRUCTIONS

Heat oven to 350. Toast English muffin on light setting. Spread 1 Tbsp of pizza sauce on each muffin half. Top with shredded cheese and 3 slices pepperoni for each half. Bake for 8 minutes. This is a great, healthy pizza fix during the week! Makes a good lunch or bedtime snack.

NUTRTION INFO

Makes 1 Serving
(One Serving)

200 calories
5 grams of fat
23 grams of carbs
3 grams of fiber
16 grams of protein

Fiesta Chicken

4 boneless skinless chicken breasts

1 ½ cups Baked Tortilla chips, crushed

1 cup 2% shredded cheddar cheese

Lime Juice

Non-stick cooking spray

INSTRUCTIONS

Grill chicken breasts on a tabletop grill or outdoor grill until no longer pink, occasionally brushing with lime juice. While chicken is cooking, heat oven to 375 and spray a 9 x 12 dish with cooking spray. Place crushed chips on bottom of dish. When chicken is cooked through, place on top of chips and sprinkle with cheese. Bake for 10 minutes or until cheese is melted. Serve with Mexi-Corn.

NUTRTION INFO

Makes 4 servings
(One Large Serving)

270 calories
10 grams of fat
18 grams of carbs
1 gram of fiber
30 grams of protein

Greek Turkey Burgers

1 Jenni-o Turkey Store frozen turkey burger

1 Joseph's Pita

1/2 cup Greek Yogurt or Plain Yogurt

1 tsp basil

1 small cucumber, sliced

1 small tomato, sliced

INSTRUCTIONS

Cook or grill turkey burger according to package instructions. Stir basil in yogurt.

Split pita, fill with cooked turkey burger, cucumbers and tomatoes.

Drizzle with yogurt or use as a dip.

NUTRTION INFO

Makes 1 serving
(One Large Serving)

310 calories
9 grams of fat
18 grams of carbs
5 grams of fiber
35 grams of protein

High Fiber Apple Cinnamon Oatmeal

1 package of Quaker High Fiber Instant Oatmeal in Cinnamon Swirl

1/2 cup Skim Milk

1 medium apple, chopped

INSTRUCTIONS

Prepare oatmeal with milk according to package directions, adding the apples before microwaving. Cook according to directions, sprinkle with a little extra cinnamon if desired.

NUTRTION INFO

Makes 1 serving
(One Large Serving)

232 calories
2 grams of fat
58 grams of carbs
15 grams of fiber
8 grams of protein

High Fiber Cottage Cheese Breakfast

1/2 cup cottage cheese

½ cup no sugar added canned peaches

1 tsp Metamucil Clear and Natural

INSTRUCTIONS

Stir fiber into cottage cheese, top with peaches. Makes a great snack too!

NUTRTION INFO

Makes 1 Serving
(One Large Serving)

175 calories
2 grams of fat
21 grams of carbs
4 grams of fiber
15 grams of protein

High Fiber Yogurt Peanut Butter Salad

1 container vanilla Fiber-One yogurt

2 tbsp PB2 powdered peanut butter

1 medium apple, chopped

INSTRUCTIONS

In a small bowl, mix yogurt and PB2. Stir in chopped apples and enjoy for breakfast or snack.

NUTRTION INFO

Makes 1 Serving
(One Large Serving)

180 calories
3 grams of fat
29 grams of carbs
11 grams of fiber
7 grams of protein

Kari's Salsa

4 ripe tomatoes

1 green pepper

1/2 a yellow onion

Juice from 1/2 a lemon

1 handful of fresh cilantro

1 garlic clove

1/2 teas sea salt

INSTRUCTIONS

Dice onion and soak in 1 cup of water. This will make the onion taste smoother. Slice the tomato and green pepper into wedges. Add to a food processor and process until diced. Put aside in a separate bowl. Dice garlic and cilantro. Rinse onion and add onion, garlic and cilantro to food processor. Process for about 5 seconds. Add onion, garlic and cilantro to tomatoes and green pepper. Roll lemon on counter to allow juices to flow and cut in half. Squeeze the juice of half the lemon into salsa and add sea salt. Chill in the refrigerator for a couple of hours or serve immediately. For a hot version, add 1 diced jalapeno, for a sweet version add ½ a diced mango.

Submitted by Kari Strunc

NUTRTION INFO

(One Large Serving)

35 calories
0 grams of fat
8 grams of carbs
2 grams of fiber
1 gram o protein

Low Carb Mexican Chicken Wrap

1 Mission low-carb tortilla

2-3 tbsp

¼ cup

1 tbsp

1 Mexi-corn

2% Shredded Mexican cheese

Light Sour Cream

Grilled Chicken Breast

INSTRUCTIONS

Grill chicken, then cut into strips, Cook mexi-corn according to instructions, Top tortilla with cheese and warm until cheese is melted, add chicken, corn, and sour cream to the tortilla then fold and enjoy!

NUTRTION INFO

Makes 1 serving
(One Large Serving)

350 calories
12 grams of fat
26 grams of carbohydrates
12 grams of fiber
37 grams of protein

Low-Fat French Toast

4 slices	Light Italian Bread
1/2 cup	Egg Beaters
1/4 cup	Skim Milk
1 tsp	Cinnamon
1 tsp	Vanilla Extract
1 tbsp	Splenda
¼ cup	Sugar Free Syrup

INSTRUCTIONS

Pre-heat griddle to medium heat, spray with non-stick spray, Beat egg beaters, vanilla, cinnamon, splenda, and milk in a small bowl, Dip top and bottom of bread in mixture and place on griddle, Cook until both sides are golden brown and top with syrup.

Great breakfast, add turkey sausage for extra protein!

¼ cup of maple syrup is 210 calories and 53 grams of sugar.

The makes a great pre-workout meal!

NUTRTION INFO

Makes 1 serving
4 Slices of French Toast & Sugar-free Syrup

265 calories
2 grams of fat
45 grams of carbohydrates
8 grams of fiber
20 grams of protein

Low-Carb & High Fiber Tortilla Strips

6 Low-Carb Tortillas

Non-stick cooking spray

Salt

INSTRUCTIONS

Using a pizza cutter, cut tortillas into ¼ inch strips. Heat oven to 375. Place tortilla strips on a baking sheet in a single layer and spray with cooking spray. Sprinkle with salt. Bake for 3 minutes, remove from oven and lightly stir up the strips, then bake for an additional 4-5 minutes until light brown. Cool and store in a gallon-sized ziplock bag. You can also use different seasonings such as cinnamon, All-Spice, Chili Powder, etc. to make different flavored strips. Enjoy on their own or with hummus, salsa or other low-fat dip.

NUTRTION INFO

110 calories
2.5 grams of fat
18 grams of carbs
11 grams of fiber
5 grams of protein

Makes 4-6 servings
(One Large Serving)

Mini Veggie Pizzas

1 Joseph's Flax Pita, halved

2 tbsp pizza sauce

4 thin slices of zucchini

1 sliced portabello mushroom

1 plum or grape tomato, diced

2% shredded mozzerella cheese

INSTRUCTIONS

Toast each pita half. Top each half with 1 Tbl of pizza sauce, zucchini, mushroom and tomato, sprinkle with 2% mozzarella cheese and bake at 350 for 8 minutes or until cheese is melted.

NUTRTION INFO

(One Large Serving)

210 calories
7 grams of fat
20 grams of carbs
7 grams of fiber
16 grams of protein

Nathan's Blueberry Muffins

1 cup whole wheat flour

1 cup wheat bran

1/2 cup pure cane sugar crystals

1 Tbsp baking powder

1/2 teas salt

1 cup skim milk

1/4 cup Egg Beater's

1/4 cup unsweetened apple sauce

1 cup frozen blueberries (do not thaw)

INSTRUCTIONS

Heat the oven to 375. Mix the flour, wheat bran, sugar, baking powder and salt in a large bowl. In a separate bowl mix the milk, egg and applesauce. Pour the milk mixture in the flour mixture and stir until combined. Stir in the blueberries. Pour the batter into 9 greased or lined muffin cups. Fill any remaining empty muffin cups 2/3's full of water to prevent pan from burning. Sprinkle extra cane sugar over the top of each muffin. Bake for about 20 minutes or until golden brown and firm to the touch. Store at room temperature for 2 days or freeze for up to 3 weeks. When freezing, wrap individually and store in plastic bag or airtight container.

Submitted by Nathan Strunc

NUTRTION INFO

Makes 12 Mufins

(One Muffin)

140 calories

1 gram of fat

26 grams of carbs

2 grams of fiber

4 grams of protein

One Pan Tacos

1lb Extra Lean Ground Turkey

2 cups water

1 Package Taco Seasoning

2 cups Minute Brown Rice, uncooked

1 cup 2% shredded Mexican Cheese

Lettuce, tomatoes, black olives to taste

INSTRUCTIONS

Brown meat in large skillet and drain. Stir in water and seasoning mix and bring to a boil. Mix in rice, top with cheese and cover. Reduce heat to low and simmer for 5 minutes. Top with tomato, lettuce, black olives as desired.

NUTRTION INFO

Makes 4 servings
(One Large Serving)

360 calories
9 grams of fat
35 grams of carbs
2 grams of fiber
37 grams of protein

Oatmeal Bran Cake

1 1/2 cups boiling water

1/2 cup rolled oats

1/2 cup whole bran cereal

1 cup white sugar

1 cup light brown sugar

1/2 cup yogurt

1/2 cup Egg Beaters

1 tsp baking soda

1 tsp ground cinnamon

1 tsp salt

1 1/2 cups all purpose flour
(One 3in x 3in square)

INSTRUCTIONS

Pour boiling water over oats and bran cereal and let stand for 10 minutes. Combine remaining ingredients and add to oat mixture. Bake at 350 for 30-40 minutes for 2, 8-9 inch cake pans or 15 minutes for muffins. Makes a great snack!

Submitted by Maria Rehlander

NUTRITION INFO

160 calories
1/2 gram of fat
36 grams of carbs
4 grams of fiber
2 grams of protein

Cakes 2: 9-inch Cakes

Peanut Butter Banana Smoothie

12oz skim milk

1 banana broken into chunks and frozen (not required but makes for a thicker smoothie)

2 tbsp PB2 powdered peanut butter

1/2 cup of Quick Cooking Oats

INSTRUCTIONS

Combine all ingredients in blender and blend until smooth.

NUTRTION INFO

Makes 1 serving
(One Large Serving)

415 calories
4 grams of fat
72 grams of carbs
8 grams of fiber
24 grams of protein

Sandra's High Fiber Strawberry Smoothie

1 single serve size container of Fiber One strawberry yogurt

1/2 cup strawberries, fresh or frozen

8oz skim milk

INSTRUCTIONS

Place all ingredients in a blender and blend until smooth.

Submitted by Sandra Carlson

NUTRTION INFO

Makes 1 serving
(One Large Serving)

170 calories
0 grams of fat
34 grams of carbs
7 grams of fiber
12 grams of protein

Low Fat Sliders

1lb 93/7 ground beef or turkey

Seasoned Salt

1 package of a dozen Sarah Lee wheat dinner rolls

Non-stick cooking spray

INSTRUCTIONS

Heat oven to 350. Spray 9 x 12 glass dish with cooking spray, press meat into dish, spreading evenly. Sprinkle with seasoned salt and bake for 18 minutes or until meat is no longer pink. Cut rolls and place one burger on each roll. Wrap remaining burgers in foil and freeze to enjoy later for a quick snack or meal. You can also try your own variety of seasonings as well and top with your favorite condiments.

NUTRTION INFO

Makes 12 serving (One Slider)

160 calories
4 grams of fat
22 grams of carbs
3 grams of fiber
12 grams of protein

Quinoa Chili

1lb 93/7 ground beef

1 medium yellow onion, diced

32 ounces stewed or crushed tomatoes

4 ounce jar of pureed carrots (baby food)

1 can Aduki beans*

1/2 cup of dried Quinoa**, prepared according to package directions before adding to chili

INSTRUCTIONS:

Cook meat on medium, add diced onion. Drain any remaining grease or blot with a paper towel. Add tomatoes and carrots and cook for 5 minutes. Add beans and prepared Quinoa, cook for additional 5 minutes. Add salt and pepper to taste. Great served with corn chips!

*Aduki beans are usually found in the health food section of your grocery store and are rich in fiber. They are a good source of iron, protein and magnesium.

**Quinoa is high in protein. It contains an almost perfect balance of all 8 essential amino acids needed for tissue development in humans.

Submitted by Lori DuBay

NUTRTION INFO

Makes 6 Servings
(One Serving)

206 calories
5 grams of fat
21 grams of carbs
5 grams of carbs
25 grams of protein

Sloppy Jose's

1lb 93/7 ground beef or ground turkey

1 package taco seasoning mix

1 can Mexicorn, divided

1/2 cup black beans, rinsed and drained

1 cup shredded 2% cheddar cheese

8 light Italian hamburger buns

INSTRUCTIONS

Cook meat in a skillet until no longer pink. Add water and taco seasoning mix according to package directions. Add ½ a can of Mexicorn and black beans and simmer for 5-7 minutes until heated through. Serve on hamburger buns and top with shredded cheese and salsa if desired. Serve additional Mexicorn on the side.

NUTRTION INFO

Makes 8 Servings

(One Sloppy Jose)

210 calories

5 grams of fat

24 grams of carbs

4 grams of fiber

17 grams of protein

Southwestern BLT Wraps

1 low-carb tortilla

2 slices center cut, or turkey, bacon

1 small tomato, sliced

1 cup lettuce, torn

1 Tbsp fat-free mayo

1 Tbsp salsa

INSTRUCTIONS

Cook bacon in microwave according to package instructions. Meanwhile, stir together mayo and salsa. Spread mayo mixture on tortilla, top with bacon, lettuce and tomato, roll-up.

NUTRTION INFO

Makes 1 Serving
(One Large Serving)

180 calories
5 grams of fat
24 grams of carbs
13 grams of fiber
12 grams of protein

Summer Salad with Chicken

1 5oz package of salad greens

1 cup of fresh strawberries, sliced

1 11oz can of mandarin oranges, drained

1 package of ready to eat chicken chunks

1/4 cup slivered or sliced almonds

1/4 cup light Raspberry Vinagrette dressing

INSTRUCTIONS

Combine all ingredients and drizzle with dressing. Serve with a Joseph's Pita on the side.

NUTRTION INFO

Makes 4 servings
(One Large Serving)

185 calories
7 grams of fat
17 grams of carbs
3 grams of fiber
15 grams of protein

Taco Salad

1lb 93/7 ground beef or ground turkey

1 package taco seasoning mix

2 cups Romaine lettuce, torn

1 cup 2% shredded Mexican cheese

1 tomato, chopped

1 2.25 oz can sliced black olives

2 low-carb tortillas

1/2 cup Daisy Light Sour Cream

2 Tbsp taco sauce

INSTRUCTIONS

Heat oven to 375. Place tortillas on a baking sheet and spray lightly with cooking spray. Bake for 4 minutes, turn, bake an additional 4 minutes or until lightly browned. Cool and break into pieces. Mix sour cream with taco sauce. Brown meat in a skillet until no longer pink. Add taco seasoning and water according to package instructions. Combine meat, tortilla pieces, lettuce, tomato, and olives. Sprinkle with cheese. Drizzle with sour cream mixture.

NUTRTION INFO

Makes 6 servings
(One Large Serving)

290 calories
10 grams of fat
25 grams of carbs
7 grams of fiber
23 grams of protein

Turkey Picadillo

1lb 93/7 ground turkey

¼ teas garlic

1 tsp cumin

1/4 tsp All Spice

8 oz tomato sauce

1/3 cup green olives

1/3 cup raisins

INSTRUCTIONS

Brown turkey until no longer pink, add garlic, cumin, all spice, tomato sauce, olives and raisins. Simmer for 10 minutes. This is very versatile and can be served a few ways or enjoyed as is. Serve in romaine leaves with brown rice, or in a low-carb torilla, or in a Joseph's pita.

NUTRTION INFO

Makes 4 Servings
(One Large Serving)

191 calories
3 grams of fat
14 grams of carbs
2 grams of fiber
27 grams of protein

Turkey Ricotta Roll-Ups

6 slices thick carved deli turkey (for meal, 3 would make a good snack)

1/2 cup part skim ricotta cheese

Italian seasoning to taste

1/4 cup Parmesean cheese

Non-stick cooking spray

INSTRUCTIONS

Heat oven to 350. Spray 2 qt baking dish with cooking spray. In a small bowl, stir together ricotta cheese and Italian seasoning. Sprinkle Parmesan cheese onto a plate. Spoon ricotta mixture evenly onto each turkey slice, then roll turkey around the cheese. Roll turkey roll-up in Parmesan and place seam-side down in the baking dish. Bake for 13 minutes or until heated through.

NUTRTION INFO

(One Large Serving)

191 calories
3 grams of fat
14 grams of carbs
2 grams of fiber
27 grams of protein

Turkey, Apple and Swiss Sandwich

3 slices shaved Deli Turkey

2 slices Light Italian Bread

1/2 an apple, thinly sliced

1 slice of reduced-fat Swiss Cheese

1 Tbl of mustard

INSTRUCTIONS

Toast each slice of Light Italian Bread and spread with mustard. Microwave apple slices for 30 seconds until slightly softened and place half the slices on the toast, top with turkey and swiss cheese, then remaining apple slices and toast. Serve the other half of the apple as a side.

NUTRITIONAL INFO

Makes 1 serving
(One Large Serving)

240 calories
2 grams of fat
27 grams of carbs
5 grams of fiber
29 grams of protein

The Spike Diet©
Quick Reference Guide

Food to Eat

- Lean Meats
- Fish
- Poultry
- Protein Powders
- Beans and Legumes
- Eggs
- Nuts
- Skim Milk
- Reduced Fat Cheese
- Vegetables
- Fruits
- Oats
- Whole Grains
- Quinoa
- Olive Oil
- Coconut Oil

Foods to Avoid

- Sugar
- White Bread
- White Pasta
- Vegetable Oil
- Butter
- Shortening
- Whole Milk
- Whole Fat Cheese
- Processed Foods
- Cereals High in Sugar
- HFCS

Protein	*Biological Value (BV)**
Whey Protein Isolates	100-159
Whole Egg	100
Milk	91
Fish	82
Beef	80
Chicken	79
Soy	74
Casein	71

**VALUES ARE APPROXIMATE*

Food	Glycemic Index
Maltose	105
Glucose	100
Sucrose	65
Honey	58
Lactose (milk)	46
Fructose (fruit)	23
Bagel	72
White Bread	70
Whole Wheat Bread	69
Sour Dough Bread	52
Sponge Cake	46
Watermelon	103
Pineapple	66
Cantaloupe	65
Banana	55
Grapes	46
Orange	44
Apple	38
Cherries	22

Sugars Grains Fruits

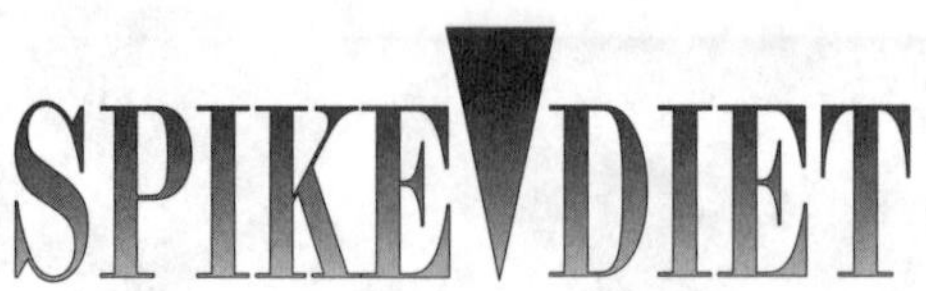

QUICK START GUIDE

Height in Inches	Weight in Pounds	Age

Harris and Benedict RMR Formula

Women: RMR=655+(4.35 x weight in pounds) + (4.7 x height in inches) - (4.7 x age in years)
Men: RMR=66+(6.23 x weight in pounds) + (12.7 x height in inches) - (6.8 x age in years)

RMR=	

Daily Resting Calories burned-High Day	RMR		X 3= Weekly Calories on a High Day
Low Day	RMR - 500		X 3= Weekly Calories on a Low Day
SPIKE DAY	RMR X 2		
Average Total Calories Burned with Activity	(TDEE)= RMR X 1.55		X 7= Weekly Calories Burned

Activity Multiplier for TDEE

Sedentary=RMR x 1.2 (little or no exercise or activity)
Lightly Active=RMR x 1.375 (exercise and activity 1-3 days/wk)
Moderately Active=RMR x 1.55 (exercise and activity 3-5 days/wk)
Very Active=RMR x 1.725 (exercise and activity 6-7 days/wk)
Extremely Active=RMR x 1.9 (daily exercise or physical job)

Total Calories Burned	Total Calories Consumed	Burned-Consumed =(Deficit)	Divide Deficit by 3500 (1lb)	Pounds lost per week

The chart below shows you a good goal of macronutrients to aim for daily based on the amount of calories you eat. The chart is for both men and women who are lifting weights 3-5 times a week.

Calories	Fat 20%	Carbs 40 %	Protein 40%
1200	27 grams	120 grams	120 grams
1500	33 grams	150 grams	150 grams
1750	39 grams	175 grams	175 grams
2000	44 grams	200 grams	200 grams
2500	56 grams	250 grams	250 grams

For the men and women who are not lifting weights, you will not need as much protein.

Calories	Fat 20%	Carbs 60 %	Protein 20%
1200	27 grams	180 grams	60 grams
1500	33 grams	225 grams	75 grams
1750	39 grams	262 grams	88 grams
2000	44 grams	300 grams	100 grams
2500	56 grams	375 grams	125 grams

Works Cited

1) http://www.shrinkyourself.com/why_diets_fail_emotional_hunger.asp

2) http://notesapps.unon.org/notesapps/unonbb.nsf/Search/2460114FAA839424432573D166?OpenDocument

3) http://www.netwellness.org/question.cfm/28525.htm

4) http://www.weightlossresources.co.uk/calories/burning_calories/starvation.htm

5) http://absoluteastronomy.com/topics/Famine_response

6) http://www.netwellness.org/uestion.cfm/64453.htm

7 http://www.bulimiahelp.org/book/restrictive-eating-studies/anselkeys%E2%80%99s-minnesota-semi-starvation-study

8) http://www.weight-loss-tips-and-secrets.com/calorie-intake.html

9) http://www.apinchofhealth.com/resources/BMR-and-calories.html

10) Earl Mindell's Peak Performance Bible, Colman, Mindell, Publisher Fireside January 4, 2001.

11) http://www.associatedcontent.com/article/371448/understanding_the_thermogenic_effects.html?cat=5

12) http://www.medicinenet.com/script/main/art.asp?articlekey=16336

13) www.diabetesnet.com/diabetes_food_diet/glycemic_index.php

14) http://www.coconutresearchcenter.org/article10612.htm

15) http://www.brighthub.com/health/diet-nutrition/article/25599.aspx

16) http://www.bmi-calculator.net/bmr-calculator/harris-benedict-equation-equation/

17) http://www.bmi-calculator.net/bmr-calculator/harris-benedict-equation/calorie-intake-to-lose-weight.php

18) http://www.ast-ss.com/matot.php

19) http://www.mikementzer.com

20) http://www.intervaltraining.net/hiit.html

The Spike Diet Daily Food and Exercise Journal's are now available at www.spikediet.com, please visit my website for more information and join the Facebook fanpage.

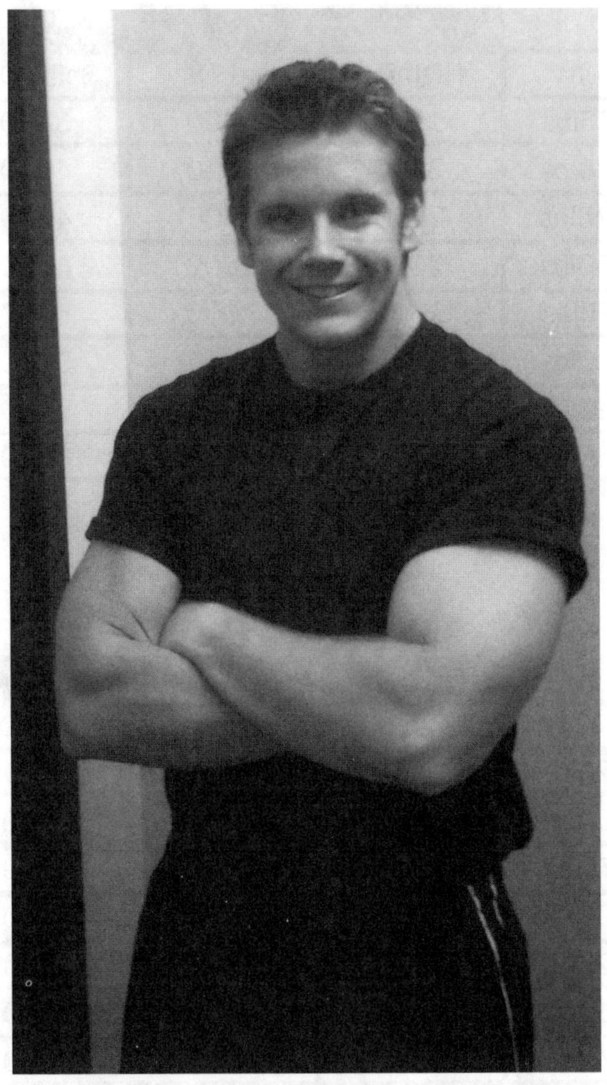

"This is not your fault, losing weight is not as simple as eating less and exercising more but it is as simple as truly believing in yourself and sticking to your commitment."

Quick Start Daily Calorie Guide

	Calorie Goal		
Men	High Day	Low Day	Spike Day
175lbs	1900	1400	3800
200lbs	2000	1500	4000
225lbs	2100	1600	4200
250lbs	2300	1800	4600
275lbs	2500	2000	5000
300lbs	2600	2100	5200
325lbs	2700	2200	5400
350lbs	2800	2300	5600

	Calorie Goal		
Women	High Day	Low Day	Spike Day
125lbs	1350	1200	2700
150lbs	1450	1200	2900
175lbs	1600	1200	3200
200lbs	1700	1200	3400
225lbs	1800	1300	3600
250lbs	1900	1400	3800
275lbs	2000	1500	4000
300lbs	2100	1600	4200

(Estimate is not as accurate as the Harris and Benedict Formula)